The Paradigm Shift in Health

Towards a Quantum Understanding of the Role of Consciousness in Health Promotion and Education

Ronald S. Laura and Amy Chapman

with Mark Hinchey

University Press of America,® Inc.
Lanham · Boulder · New York · Toronto · Plymouth, UK

4501 Forbes Boulevard
Suite 200
Lanham, Maryland 20706
UPA Acquisitions Department (301) 459-3366

Estover Road
Plymouth PL6 7PY
United Kingdom

Printed in the United States of America
British Library Cataloging in Publication Information Available

Library of Congress Control Number: 2009922305
ISBN-13: 978-0-7618-4556-0 (paperback : alk. paper)
ISBN-10: 0-7618-4556-9 (paperback : alk. paper)
eISBN-13: 978-0-7618-4557-7
eISBN-10: 0-7618-4557-7

™ The paper used in this publication meets the minimum requirements of American National Standard for Information Sciences—Permanence of Paper for Printed Library Materials, ANSI Z39.48—1984

Dedications

No book is written in isolation, and whenever a book is co-authored to fruition, as this one has been, an almost miraculous partnership of mind and emotional commitment to the task emerge almost ineluctably. The arduous and sometimes tedious burdens of gathering and analysing research data, books, articles, conference papers and the like can be almost overwhelming, given the persistent pressure to translate such effort into a written form sufficient to materialising almost magically as a manuscript for publication. It would be remiss of me then not to thank abundantly and dedicate this book to my co-author, Ms Amy Chapman, for the prodigious effort she has made to tolerate my creative eccentricities, along with two years of intense dialogue and revision of script. Indeed, in this case, I do so graciously knowing that the intellectual torch one hopes to pass to the hands of one's students burns ever more brightly and will indeed be transferred to others as part of the relentless chain of learning and teaching in which we engage. Congratulations, Ms Chapman on our joint book.

Ronald. S Laura

To my family - Mum, Dad and Penny. I dedicate this book to you in honour of our precious gift of family. May the publishing of this book inspire in us a renewed quest for the elusive bounty of health and happiness. We have learnt first hand that whilst the journey for health and happiness may be arduous, the price we pay for not searching is infinitely greater. Also, to my co-author, Ron, my teacher, mentor and friend. I can never repay your kindness and wisdom. I will strive always to be a better teacher and person because of you. Thank you for showing me that in the midst of busy and complicated lives we should never be too busy to nurture the values that make life really living.

Amy Chapman

I would like to thank my wife Lindsay and our two beautiful children for their love and support during my contribution to this book. Second, I would like to extend my appreciation to Ron and Amy for the opportunity given to me to come on board as a co-author, an experience I have thoroughly enjoyed. Finally, I would like to thank you for purchasing a copy of this book, with the hope that you will be further enriched on you journey towards wholeness.

Mark Hinchey

Table of Contents

Introduction

We are in the midst of a revolutionary philosophical breakthrough in our understanding of the nature of reality and a new way of thinking about the world, whose implications are momentous for how we conceive of the human body and its capacity for what we have called elsewhere, 'integrated well-being'.[1]

The conceptual dimensions of this new vision of the world has certain of its metaphysical roots in eastern religions, one of the best know of which is the healing tradition of India called *Ayurveda.* The etymology of the word 'Ayurveda' derives from two distinct words drawn together as one ideational form from the Sanskrit. The first Sanskrit root word is *Ayus*, meaning 'life', and the second root word is *Veda* which conveys in English the idea of 'knowledge'. 'Life knowledge' or the 'science of life', as it is more popularly called, is sponsored on the assumption that an energy force known as *Prana* is channeled through the body like a wind, called *Vata,* one of the life defining principles or doshas. Vata is depicted as being responsible for the metabolic regulation of five seemingly discrete but systematically related networks. The life-energy force which sustains the physical body is termed *Prana Vata*. In so far as it provides the source of energy for the living body and consolidates the biological functions for the remaining Vata, namely circulation, digestion, excretion and cognitive capabilities including intellect, memory, speech, etc. Prana Vata is reckoned to be the primary regulator of importance upon which the others are dependent. When Prana Vata is out of balance, the Vata which regulate the other major bodily functions will be thus also be disrupted. This being so, Ayurveda places considerable emphasis, both from a preventative perspective and from a healing one, upon the relationship between health maintenance and the balanced function of Prana Vada. The success enjoyed by Ayurvedic medicine has in recent years been brought to public attention in the western world through the growing practice of meditation and the educational infrastructure surrounding it. In addition practitioners of Ayurvedic medicine such as Deepak Chopra have done much to familiarize those seeking alternative approaches to medicine with Ayurvedic traditions in medicine, largely through books, articles, lectures, television and other media presentations. Similar interest has been shown in varying degrees to Chi Cong, Reiki and even psychic healing.

The revolutionary breakthrough with which we shall be concerned in this book acknowledges the valuable contribution that Ayurvedic medicine and certain of its cognate wholistic alternatives are capable of making to the health and medical possibilities and healing practices. None the less, there remains a theoretical hiatus between the pragmatics of praxis and the philosophical foundations required to articulate them. This is especially a problem concerning the fact that a deep tension continues to exist between these alternative approaches and conventional medicine. This is to some extent understandable in that the philosophical foundations of conventional medicine, however myopic and dogmatically delimiting they might be, are theoretically articulated very well. Whether one chooses to accept it or not, the bioreductionist philosophical framework of interpretation is extremely well enunciated, and it is palpably clear that without considerable revision there is no place for the 'wind-like' energy or life force of *Prana Vada* to be accommodated. Nor does how Prana Vada functions from within the framework of Ayurvedic medicine reveal a sufficiently well articulated philosophical foundation for the proponents of conventional medicine to be persuaded of even the possibility of its theoretical validity. Lest we be misunderstood, it is imperative to make clear that in admitting this difficultly, we are not suggesting that Pranic healing does in fact work; the point is that no adequate philosophical articulation has yet been provided for wholistic approaches to medicine which might serve to convince a conventional practitioner as to why such alternatives can at least in principle be said to work.

Lamentably, the term "wholism" in the conventional medical context immediately conjures the image of exotic therapies and bizarre alternatives to the standard techniques of orthodox medicine. There is little doubt that wholistic medicine has come to encompass a wide array of medical procedures such as homeopathy, acupressure, acupuncture, reflexology, iridology, Rolfing, the Alexander technique, Lomi body work, the Feldenkrais method, bioenergetic analysis, polarity therapy, chelation therapy, and visualization therapy, to name only a few. The reaction against wholistic medical practices has in some circles been resoundingly vituperative and condemnatory. Typical of the cynical response to wholism, Glymour and Stalker write, "Wholistic medicine is pabulum of common sense and nonsense offered by cranks and quacks and failed pedants who share an attachment to magic and an animosity to reason."[2] It is not our purpose as such to defend any of the specific wholistic healing practices alluded to above, though we are confident that several of them clearly admit of defense. We do contend, however, that it is a mistake to condemn wholistic philosophy of medicine simply on the basis of the *conventional* unacceptability of a specific wholistic health or medical practice. Nor do we claim for wholistic health the liberating originality which other supporters might urge in its defense.

The split between conventional and alternative approaches to medicine can be traced back to at least the late 1700s, when Samuel Hahnemann proposed homeopathy (the idea that every disease can be cured by the specific drug capable of creating a similar set of symptoms) as an alternative to conventional techniques. [3] None the less, the wholistic philosophy of medicine emerges from the Hippocratic tradition of medicine itself, and its renewed emphasis merely restores to medicine an approach which was there from its inception, and education has been an important facet of its delivery. That people can become actively involved as *informed* participants in the process of primary health care presupposes an educational program which extends the intellectual imagination beyond the domain of conventional health matters. Such education must be capable of reflecting the relevant personal, social, cultural, and political characteristics which contribute uniquely to the health problems peculiar to specific countries and the more pervasive cultural traditions of which they may form a part. The idea of approaching the goal of integrated well-being with a scientific model of medicine that fails to acknowledge the salient role in health played by environmental factors, emotional factors, and cultural beliefs is naïve and misguided.

Within this framework of integrative approach certain of the philosophical assumptions which underpin the conventional approach to health education must themselves be reconceptualized. The belief that all health problems can be explained in conventional medical terms hides the truth that at least some of the problems which resist such explanation constitute by their very nature a challenge to the conventional view of medicine. One persistent objection to alternative medical therapies has been that "for none of the theories considered is there firm evidence that the therapy is generally more effective than a credible placebo in relieving any sort of clinical problem or in producing any kind of therapeutic benefit." [4] Notice that even if this charge were true, it presupposes that the placebo affect is a "nuisance variable" or "psychological phenomenon" of no genuine therapeutic interest and thus outside the remit of somatic medicine. Conventional medicine has dealt with the placebo effect, in other words, by excluding it or by regarding it as an impertinent impostor and a destructive distraction from the science of into "real" therapeutics.

The fact that conventional medicine has systematically excluded or ignored the placebo effect is especially revealing when we acknowledge that the research which has been done on placebos establishes convincingly that they are a powerful therapeutic tool, not to be neglected. In a provocative article by Linnie Price, studies are reported which document that efficacy of the placebo effect. [5] In one study by Bourne, placebos were show to be effective in the relief of cough, mood changes, headache, seasickness, status asthmaticus, depression, hypertension, and even angina pectoris. In studies undertaken by Singer and Hurwitz placebos were found to be effective in lowering blood sugar levels in diabetics. Klopfer has demonstrated that placebos can be used to shrink tumors in patients with lymphosarcoma, while Beecher has shown the use of placebos in providing significant relief in patients suffering from postoperative pain. Vinar discovered the addictive effect of placebos, showing that they exhibit a number of the formal traits associated with drug dependency, including the need for increased dosage and withdrawal symptoms upon sudden deprivation of medication. Lasagna et al. have found that placebos simulate the effects produced by 'active' pharmacological agents, and Jospe has shown that they can function as nocebos, exhibiting a wide variety of *unpleasant* side-effects. In a study undertaken by Wolf and Pinsky, some patients who were cured of anxiety and tension by ingesting placebos exhibited a range of side-effects such as epigastric pain, urticaria, and angioneurotic oedema of the lips. This report seems all the more remarkable once we are cognizant of the fact that the side-effects produced by the placebo mimic the side-effects of the active drugs which the patient would otherwise have taken for the condition. Equally intriguing is a study undertaken by Gammer and Allen which demonstrated that not only are "real" effects produced when subjects believe that a placebo is a "real" drug, but believe that a real drug is a placebo similarly produces a lack of effect.

One purpose of this protracted discussion of the placebo effect is to highlight the fact that the standard objection to alternative wholistic practices on the ground that they are no more effective than a placebo depends upon the very conventional interpretation of placebos which such practices serve by their very nature to challenge. As Price aptly puts it:

> Medicine's chosen self location in science necessitates the exclusion of non-observable phenomena . . . from its knowledge; they cannot simply be incorporated. They are variable and unpredictable in a way that the objects of natural science are not (although the subjects of social science are). Yet their existence, and extent, renders equivocal that very scientific knowledge that excludes them, just as subjectivity and meaning have daunted sociologists' attempts to explain the social world via the scientific canons of positivism. Medicine has dealt with the placebo effect in the only way its paradigm logically permits---exclusion. To accept the implications of the placebo effect would be to challenge the claims to truth of all medical knowledge: it would necessitate a paradigmatic revolution of untold proportions. The placebo effect demonstrates that illness and cure properly belong in the social, not the natural world. [6]

The second reason for this protracted discussion of the 'placebo effect' is that the psychosomantic processes which partly define this intriguing phenomenon provide a significant starting place for the elaboration of the revolutionary paradigm of quantum healing under consideration here. On the quantum vision of healing presently being postulated, the idea that illness can be construed simply as a manifestation of any of a variety of purely physiological disruptions to the established harmony of the human organism is fundamentally misguided. Almost without exception neither sickness nor disease can be reduced entirely to bodily physics. The web of energetic field which characterizes quantum consciousness is so seamlessly interwoven with the physical universe of the bodily function that mind / body duality collapses, in some ways not unlike the collapse of a wave function. The disjunction between mind and body is spurious. The mind and body are not two separate things; they are complementary facets of one and the same thing: a living, vital human being. The two concepts are not coterminous in extension, but they are so inextricably connected that they are more like two sides of the same coin. To put it differently, every cell in the body is what we shall call a 'field - dimension' of the energy of the mind. This being so, every cell in the body is inextricably linked with every thought we think, and thus every cell in the body is systematically informed and defined not only physically but genetically. Although the concept may be difficult to fathom, the deepest truth about the nature of our being is that we are the co-authors of our own destiny and our health.

Whether illness and cure properly belong in the social and not the natural world is a question which evinces a misunderstanding. What we seek to provide instead is a framework of wholistic interpretation sufficiently comprehensive to show that both social and natural phenomena can adequately and more richly be explained within it. Our contention is that the conventional framework of understanding is too limited to do justice to either social or natural phenomena, and thus that any philosophy of health education which derives from it will be equally restricted in scope. The crisis in health care cannot be resolved simply through the noble process of educating for health if the philosophy of health education which is its source is also in crisis. It is our view that the crisis in health care derives from a misguided philosophy of health which is reflected in the hidden agenda of medical science itself. The argument for the mosaic of conceptual relations which connects medical science on the one hand and the philosophical assumptions underpinning health education on the other will constitute a substantial portion of the argument of the book, and a brief discussion of its subtlety may not be amiss here.

Whether we like it or not, all human beings are now affected by science and its products. Scientific technology, for example, has shaped the nature of our industries and economies, informed the goals and patterns of international relations, and determined in large part even the way in which we spend our leisure time. Many of these effects are obvious but some are not. We have used science to transform the world in which we live, but we have ourselves been transformed in the process. Science, or what pretends to be science, has shaped not only the concepts and categories by way of which we see the world; it has informed and oriented the concepts and categories in respect of which we see ourselves and the values we hold. Not even the institution of education has been left untainted by its ubiquitous hand. Science has in its own inimitable way come to direct much of the intellectual traffic in our halls of learning.

What we have regarded traditionally as real and how we go about investigating reality are circumscribed by the framework of scientific enquiry within which both the concept of reality and the procedures for its appropriate investigation are implicitly defined. In this regard, it will be argued that our view of reality and the methodology we employ to define it have profoundly influenced and continue to influence and delimit our basic understanding of health education. Despite protestations to the contrary, the science which has come to dominate the western world-view is not just science *per se*; it is a particular philosophy of science.

A different problem then arises for conventional medicine in regard to the parameters of its own epistemological efficacy. The issue here is that its philosophical foundations are so well articulated that it not only fails to explain but actually rejects the possibility in principle that a particular technique works, that is, is not a coincidental outcome or a consequence of placebo influences, if no determinate causal conditions obtain which admit of repeatable test. In this case a treatment which might actually be working will be rendered inexplicable or rejected out of hand, simply because its analysis fails to satisfy the determinist causal cannons of theoretical legitimation.

The distinction we make here is of paramount importance to the thesis we propose. The notion of science as a method of open enquiry which is capable of being critically reflective about its own assumptions and hidden values is a notion of science that we *accept* and try to *defend* throughout this book. In this regard we are not 'anti scientific.' The problem is that not all science *is* science of this kind. When the *idea*l of science easily becomes entwined with the sociocultural modes and institutional philosophies which serve as the vehicle for its expression, science becomes both political and philosophical. This is why science so easily degenerates into *scientism*, for it often enshrines covertly a particular political or philosophical framework which serves to delimit its capacity for critical reflection. Scientism is thus science which has lost the power to be subversive. Our aim in this book is not to urge that medicine should become less scientific, but to show that it is less scientific than it could be because it is more 'scientistic' than it should be. Medicine is not itself a science, but it relies upon science as the source of the knowledge which it applies in the service of healing. The reliability of medicine depends upon the reliability of the source of knowledge which informs it. Our claim is that the assumptions upon which scientism rests are unreliable and that conventional medicine is less reliable than it could be for the scientism which pervades it.

Two particular philosophical dispositions which have shaped medical scientism will concern us here. There is first the Newtonian view of the world as a kind of machine which consists of independent and separate parts into which it can be exhaustively analyzed. The mechanistic paradigm has become fossilized into a metaphysical postulate. Within the mechanist paradigm the human organism is construed on the model of a machine, and the doctor is regarded as a biological engineer who fixes the parts of the machine when they break down. In their defense of this paradigm Glymour and Stalker write: "The practice of medicine in the United States and in other industrialized nations is a form of consultant engineering. The subjects are people rather than bridges, but in many respects the professions of medicine and engineering are alike." [7] The direction of accepted research is oriented around the Newtonian paradigm, and though mechanism and reductionism are not to be confused, mechanism provides a rationale for a reductionist methodology of science capable of analyzing the whole of nature into the fundamental constituents alleged to determine causally its overall behavior.

Within medicine the methodology of scientific analysis has come to be known as "bioreductionism" and its impact upon health education has been staggering. Bioreductionism is the second philosophical disposition of scientism with which we will be concerned, and it has given rise to assumptions and attitudes about the nature of the body, the diseases which afflict it, and the kind of treatment appropriate to it. Coupled with the mechanist assumption that the body is a machine which from time to time malfunctions, bioreductionism ensures that the role of the doctor and the orientation of medical practice are decidedly interventionist. Not unlike an engineer repairing a faulty structure, conventional medicine is geared to intervene on behalf of the patient to repair the faulty machine.

Reductionism in medicine has also influenced the conventional interpretation of disease. The idea is that disease admits of reduction to a specific microorganism which is its cause. The temptation to suppose that health professionals should thus conduct the fight against disease by intervening on the body's behalf to destroy the invading germs in respect of which the body shows insufficient resistance, or no resistance at all, has proved to be irresistible. This being so, it is hardly surprising to find that the purported link between particular diseases and the specific microbes which caused them was quickly crystallized into a working hypothesis called the "theory of specific etiology." Having a profound influence upon the philosophy and practice of medicine, the doctrine of specific etiology reinforced the reductionist inclination to regard malfunctions of the human body as explicable causally by reference to the malfunction of a single bodily mechanism. Inasmuch as different diseases defined specific malfunctions, the interventionist approach depended upon classifying diseases in such a way that one could deduce from the classification the nature of the antipathogenic agents required to rectify the malfunction. Medical intervention was thus seen to restore a person to health by eradicating the discrete disease entities which were defined almost invariably in biochemical or biophysical terms, correlating in turn with the symptoms and other signs of a particular illness. On the bioreductionist model the concept of health was thereby construed as the absence of disease, and thus the thrust of medical research came to focus on the extirpation and control of the microorganisms which cause disease.

With the rise of a more sophisticated medical technology, medical scientism strengthened its hold on the healing traditions of the western medical world. Technological innovations such as the X-ray, the electrocardiogram, and the electroencephalogram afforded the doctor a rich arsenal of mysterious reductionist weapons to combat disease at the level of the microbe. Focus upon the microorganisms causally responsible for physiological deviations led also to a new awareness of the connection between bacteria and infection. Indeed, it was in large part the introduction of aseptic surgical procedures, in conjunction with advances in general anesthesiology, which served to ensure the success and determine the crucial part surgery would play in the implementation of the bioreductionist medical scenario. Armed with the scalpel and an impressive array of "wonder drugs" (essentially microbes designed to do battle with other microbes) modern medical science had at its disposal a growing technology of ultimate intervention.

Sponsored on the assumption that functional disturbances in the "human machine" can be traced in large part to the specific disease entities which are their source, the technology of medical science ensured that if these entities cannot be controlled or killed by other microbes, they can ultimately be eliminated by being cut out. In certain cases, what is cut out (e.g., the heart or a kidney) can be replaced by a "healthier" substitute. In this regard surgery represents a truly revolutionary dimension of the interventionist approach - surgical intervention entails not only the repair but the reconstruction of the human body. The process of intervening on behalf of the living machine culminates in either repairing or changing its parts when they can no longer be "fixed."

Despite a number of recent challenges to the traditional medical model of disease, the reductionist trend in biomedical science has continued largely unabated. Contemporary medical research is still preoccupied primarily by one aspect of the process of disease, i.e., the study of biological phenomena at the cellular and molecular level. The scientific basis of medicine *thus construed* derives from a limited understanding of the nature of biological phenomena in general. In the end, the so-called scientific view of medicine reflects only a partial view of science. One reason why it is so difficult to disabuse ourselves of the conventional concepts of health and disease is that the medical scientism from which they derive has also been used as the criterion to judge their worth. This is why the appeal to the conventional framework of medicine provides little assistance in attempting to redefine the concepts of health and disease, and it is here that we are brought full circle to the hidden agenda of education.

Since the conversion of medicine from a religious to a scientific persuasion, its apostasy has almost always been advertised as a virtue. The temptation has been to think that science has legitimated medicine, transforming its practitioners into technological giants. One need not diminish the achievements of technology to charge that the giants of reductionist medicine are blinded giants. That medicine has defected from religion to science has been reckoned to liberate medicine from irrelevant treatise and religious dogma, a freedom in respect of which medicine has long been jubilantly aware. One consequence of which medicine seems to have been less aware, however, is the extent to which its commitment to and identification with science has demanded an unwilling allegiance to an institutional and limited view of science which is itself dogmatic and blinding. It is a measure of the power of the myth of scientism that we generally take for granted that scientific technology has transformed our world and our perception of it for the better. We rely upon science to teach us about the world and about ourselves because we believe science is reliable and produces the best results. The transformation science affects makes things better - so we are told - because it is science that is the best way of doing things. It is part of our aim in this book to show that while there is much about this view of science which is attractive, the attraction is meretricious when the view is generalized and science degenerates into scientism.

The power of science as a tool for discovery and exploration within medicine is not of course to be denied. The success of bioreductionism has in certain respects been spectacular. Yet even the major triumphs of modern medicine betray the shortcomings of the philosophical framework which inspires them. Consider, for example, how the bioreductionist approach has led to the profligate use of drugs in the treatment of illness. While we have no wish to suggest that drugs are without medical value, it seems to us clear that their value has been enormously exaggerated and their side-effects woefully neglected. It has been pointed out that in the United States and the United Kingdom from 50 to 80 percent of adults swallow a medically prescribed drug every twenty-four to thirty-six hours. In addition, the analgesic aspirin is consumed at the rate of approximately 20,000 tons per year in the United States alone, thereby providing an annual intake of some 225 tablets per person. The sales of well-known psychoactive drugs such as Valium, Librium, and Miltown have soared at an unprecedented rate with 100 million prescriptions written each year. [8]

The bioreductionist search for a "magic bullet" perpetuates the use of such drugs, despite the fact that there exists considerable evidence to show that their staggering consumption is harmful. Aspirin, for instance, has been definitively linked with gastrointestinal bleeding and genitourinary pathology. Drugs such as Librium and Valium are known to be addictive, capable of producing severe withdrawal symptoms, depending upon the dosage taken, duration of consumption, and the individual. The greater the potency of the drug, moreover, the greater the potential for its harmful side-effects. The group of powerful tranquilizers known as "phenothiazines" has been relied upon heavily in the treatment of schizophrenia, though these drugs produce side-effects which include hepatitis, leukopenia, temporary musculoskeletal abnormalities, and dose-dependent impotence, not to mention tardive dyskinesia, a condition of movement disorder which is sometimes irreversible. When taken unwittingly in combination with food coloring or even with the residue of insecticides which permeate our fruits, vegetables, meats, fish, and all too often our water, certain drugs become mutilating and mutagenic. Antibiotics, notwithstanding their value in the rapid alleviation of infection and pain, have been shown to upset the body's normal bacterial flora, thereby allowing more resistant organisms to proliferate and induce superinfection. The disastrous side-effects of the drug thalidomide have been so widely publicized that to do more than cite the example here would be fatuous.

When all is said, it will in the course of the book become clear that the unbridled reliance upon drugs is just one example of a cultural ritual deriving from the reductio-mechanist tradition in medicine, a ritual whose long-term contribution to health is decidedly questionable. The etymology of the word "drug" reveals an ambiguity in this connection which is instructive. The Greeks had only one word for "drug" (i.e., *pharmakon*), and it was possessed of a double meaning, signifying both the power to *cure* and the power to *kill.* The pharmaceutical industry represents one of the dominant institutional manifestations of the bioreductionist approach to medicine, and its continued existence and exponential growth cannot be explained adequately by reference solely to its success.

Now ranked as one of the largest industries in the western world, its profit margin in the U.S. is largely dependent upon its marketing and advertising programs with the American Medical Association, in respect of which it has developed somewhat incestuous ties. The industry's central policy-making body in the U.S. is the Pharmaceutical Manufacturers Association, and it so happens that the most substantial periodical of the A.M.A. is the *Journal of the American Medical Association* (JAMA) which has in recent decades become progressively dominated by the promotion interests of the pharmaceutical industry. The uncomfortably close relationship alluded to here is not an anomaly peculiar to the JAMA. It has been noted by other writers that advertising accounts with drug companies provide approximately half the income emanating from advertising for the majority of medical journals. Within this context of the financial dependence of professional medical journals on the pharmaceutical industry, it is not unusual for conflicts of interests to arise in respect of editorial policy. Suffice it to say here that the dominant role which drugs play in contemporary medicine is not a consequence simply of their medical efficacy. Their purported value for the process of healing is promulgated as part of the myth of medical scientism.

Just as bioreductionism is only a partial picture of the biological organization of the human system, so the use of drugs in conventional medicine supplies only a partial picture of the process of healing. What is needed is not a more comprehensive account of healing in bioreductionist terms, but a comprehensive challenge to the bioreductionist framework out of which the partial pictures emerge. It is thus a gross misconception to suppose that the more "scientific" and "technological" we make medicine - either in terms of the drugs we synthesize or the surgical procedures we devise - the better it will be. In this regard the educational appeal in the Declaration of Alma-Ata is naïve, for the appeal is unwittingly to the *scientism* of our times. Conventional science has been institutionalized as the science of reductionism, and the most significant single institutional vehicle for its expression and propagation has been our schools. Indeed, it is a central contention of this book that conventional science is permeated by a scientism that currently figures as the state-sanctioned religion of our times, and that our schools and universities have in numerous ways allowed themselves to become the servants of its ideology. The authority of the church has been superseded by the state-sanctioned authority of conventional science, and religious revelation has been replaced by scientism.

Scientism is incapable of proving a comprehensive methodology for medicine because the philosophical assumptions which underpin it are self-stultifying. The result of the alliance between bioreductionism and medicine has been to fragment medical knowledge on the one hand, while narrowing the scope of health education on the other. Conventional science can no longer be regarded unequivocally as the fountain of medical knowledge, for the waters of reductionist philosophy have become stagnant. Medical scientism has so rigidly proscribed its limits in reductionist terms that the investigations which depend upon those terms lead not so much to open discovery as to a closed metaphysical perspective in virtue of which discovery is itself defined. The conceptual boundaries in respect of which the intellectual imagination deserves most to be enhanced and stimulated is the very point at which the methodology of conventional medical science now ensures that it is diminished. The imposition of dogmatic limits upon the intellectual imagination is, wherever it is found - be it in religion or in science - inimical to the task of genuine understanding and knowledge.

In the history of the confrontation between science and religion, the heresy of science served to expose the dogmatism of religion, and we believe that religion is better for the scandal. In the present work our aim is partly to expose the dogmatism of conventional medicine as a form of scientism and to determine the extent to which the current state of health education has been perverted by an uncritical acceptance of these dogmas. We will be concerned to show that reductionist medicine has proved to be a valuable but incomplete foundation upon which to erect the edifice of health education, and we believe that, not unlike dogmatic religion, it will benefit from the scandal of its epistemic credibility.

Putting the matter in this way makes it easier to appreciate the purpose and importance of this book. The central task we have set ourselves is to show that certain theoretical insights from quantum philosophy can be elaborated in such a way that they provide the basis of radically different and far more comprehensive paradigm of healing than has to date been afforded. As a consequence, 'The Paradigm Shift' serves to provide the philosophical enunciation lacking in the context of certain alternative healing traditions such as Ayurvedic medicine, while also challenging and reconceptualizing the epistemological presumptions of conventional medicine regarding the nature of the human body and the potential role which can be played by consciousness in the unfolding of integrated well-being. We call this phenomenon 'affective quantum resonance', and it is based upon the application of the quantum theory that reality and thus the human body behave far more like energy fields than solid matter. The notion that the human body is an energy field represents a significant departure from the conventional medical view of the body as a machine.

In the first chapter of the book we provide a brief historical account of the genesis of reductionist medical science. We try to show how medicine's progressive reliance upon a particular philosophical tradition within science has led unwittingly and almost imperceptibly to the development of medical scientism. We contend that the reductionist methodology embodied in medical scientism has ultimately diminished rather than enlarged the domain of medical understanding and health care. In Chapter 2 we are concerned to illustrate the extent to which reductionist medicine has initiated a crisis within medicine of staggering proportions. Contrary to the conventional wisdom, we argue that the contemporary medical tradition has done far less to advance the health of the community than we have been led to believe. Despite the eradication of many infectious diseases and a considerable decrease in infant mortality (neither of which can be attributed directly to medical science) we are not as a society healthier. Coupled with the high cost of medical care and the invidious side-effects of many conventional medical treatments, the stage has been set, we submit, for a new emphasis within the contemporary medical tradition, an emphasis which reflects a more comprehensive philosophy of nature than the reductionist orientation of medical scientism permits.

Chapter 3 is concerned largely with exploring the traditional definitions of health and disease. We observe that inasmuch as modern medical science adheres to a limited view of biology which is quantitative and reductionistically orientated, the concept of health as the absence of disease unsurprisingly reflects the impoverished philosophy of medical scientism which underpins it. In light of this, we consider the systems view of life as providing an alternative and wholisitc perspective on health. Given a wholistic universe of dynamic interrelations and seamless interconnections, it turns out that all healing is ultimately *self-healing* and all self-healing is ultimately *universal* healing. In a radical sense, the notion that "to heal is to make whole" is recast as having cosmic significance, for health and disease are themselves seen as part of the process whereby nature reorganizes itself into modes of greater complexity. Knowing how to participate in nature is enfolded into the whole of nature and vice versa. The concepts of disease and health are at once profoundly personal and profoundly ecological.

Chapter 4 is devoted to the analysis and integration of some of the sociocultural and ecological contexts which condition health and disease. We try to show the extent to which wholistic epistemology makes it easier to identify those facets of our lifestyle which are inimical to good health. Here our theory of transformative subjugation and the epistemology of power are introduced to account for the alarming rate at which modern society is systematically transforming our world of living things into increasing inert and dead things.

This theory here assists to explain the customary degradation of our food supply. We explore just some of the health problems associated with processed and artificial foods and the impact on health of the application of chemical technology to our municipal water supplies, with particular reference to the chlorination and fluoridation programs. Consideration is also given to other stress factors affecting health which derive from our contemporary lifestyle.

In Chapter 5 the concept of *primary health care* is reviewed and concluded to be a sound method for achieving the goal of health for all. Primary health care has as its basic tenet the involvement and participation of people in all aspects of their health care. In addition to this, primary health care aims at utilizing local resources to the fullest extent and is not necessarily dependent on technical interventionist practices. Rather it is based on the will and motivation of the community which jointly shares the responsibility for care. Primary health care is not intended to replace or even to compete with modern medicine but rather to act as an adjunct to it in order that the facilities of hospitals and clinics equipped to handle more complicated illnesses which do require intervention may be better utilized. Nonetheless, primary health care, properly conceived, generates reflection on the theory and practice of the dominant mode of modern medicine.

Primary health care is intended to act at the interface of the community and the professional medical services. It recognizes that many health related problems are the responsibility of the people and accepts that the people can be educated to cope with the problems which are theirs. The rationale for primary health care arises from a spirit of social justice and lends credence to the notions of rights and reciprocal responsibility or duty. The concept of *justice* and the notions of reciprocal *responsibility* are reviewed in this light, as such concepts are central to and assist the elucidation of the claim that health care is a right of the people.

In fostering individual responsibility for health, it is of the utmost importance that education programs do not degenerate into *victim-blaming* exercises. By distinguishing between health education and education for health, we hope to show that it is possible to avoid the practice of victim-blaming.

Chapter 6 is concerned to review some of the major programs undertaken during the past decade in relation to health education. Our examination reveals that the primary focus of health education has been upon the promotion of an increase in *knowledge,* postulated on the assumption that increased knowledge would lead to *attitudinal* changes and in turn to a change in *behavior* on the part of an individual or group. It was assumed further that behavioral changes would lead to an improvement in the health status of the community. Representative rather than exhaustive as they may well be, studies reveal that the demonstrated increase in health knowledge lead neither to changes in attitude nor to changes in behavior. Even in those studies which did report some small success in increased knowledge leading to attitude change, the actual health status of the individuals or groups did not improve significantly.

In light of these findings we contend that it is necessary to explore an approach to education for health which is more wholistic in orientation than its predecessors. In this regard, we examine a model proposed by Frankena which we believe can be enlisted in the service of health education. Previous models of health education have not been comprehensively based and in particular have not addressed satisfactorily the normative and factual premises which are peculiar to health education. This being so, the theory and practice of education for health have not been presented as a unified whole, but rather as a divided or fragmented program in which the practitioners too easily lose confidence because they cannot discern an adequate conception of the global purpose of education for health.

In Chapters 7 and 8 of the book we consider an alternative to the reductiomechanist paradigm of medical science. Drawing upon recent developments in the philosophy of science and quantum mechanics, we argue for a wholistic epistemology of medicine capable of supporting the non-reductionist theory of health education to be built upon it. Arguing that a more decisive and radical transition in health education is possible by rooting out reductionism at a level much deeper than the causal theory of disease, we try to establish a fundamental relationship between health and the categories by virtue of which we conceptualize the world around us. On the assumption that there is now sufficient evidence from quantum mechanics to show that the universe is one seamless and undivided web of cosmic connections, we try to give new sense to the notion that "to heal is to make whole". On the view we all defend, health is a truly universal phenomenon and not a process which can be understood independently of the bond which ties all living things to each other and to the earth. The fundamental interdependency to which recent developments in quantum physics allude inspires a profound paradigm shift in the covert value-orientation which underpins even the traditional theory of knowledge. In our futile efforts to detach ourselves from nature to achieve a neutral perspective from which to view it, we inadvertently sever the relationship of basic bonding to nature which ultimately defines the conditions of health on earth. Rather than sensing our oneness with nature, we see ourselves as distinct from it, and we are thus disposed to employ the faculty of human consciousness to dominate and control it. The more detached and removed we become from nature, the easier it is to assume a posture of exploitation towards it. By way of the reductionist-mechanist orientation of conventional science, we have reinforced the view that inasmuch as the world is a machine, it is appropriate to investigate it and all that it contains in the impersonal way we would investigate a machine. In the process of dividing the whole cosmos into its parts and its parts into even smaller parts, we have robbed nature of the very elements of identity which generate respect for and a moral response to what we find there. Having reduced all living things to genetic compilations of the chemical DNA, for example, we feel less contrite of heart and have little or no sense of moral conscience in manipulating living things, for the things we see ourselves manipulating are the chemical building-blocks out if which living things are made, *not* the things themselves. We contrive to make ourselves morally exempt, for we can do no wrong to these things which by our own doing have no identity. The reductio-mechanist paradigm of medical scientism, construed in value terms, represents an institutionalized process by virtue of which the systematic degradation of nature's identity is affected by reducing the whole of nature to its parts.

Having regarded ourselves as separate from nature, we have evolved a theory of knowledge which is tantamount to a theory of *power* over nature. The desire for mastery of the environment, coupled with our desire to achieve objectivity by detaching ourselves from it, has led to the evolution of a conceptual marriage between knowledge and conventional science which has served to maximize our expropriation of the Earth's resources, while minimizing the time and effort devoted to the task. The biography of the growth of knowledge thus betrays our insatiable appetite for *power*. We have sought total mastery and control over the environment, and we have developed a theory of knowledge and a tradition of science to enshrine it which guarantees the exploitation of nature in consequence. We have in essence institutionalized a lifestyle, motivated by an attitude towards the Earth, which has proven to be inimical to the advancement of health. In this sense, it could plausible be said that disease and illness are manifestations of the human psyche and the collective unconscious. In our lust for power it is we who must in the end take responsibility for the stockpiles of nuclear and other weapons of destruction, for the decimation of our forests and the concomitant disruption of countless ecological systems of delicate balance, for the continual pollution of the air and the chemical poisoning of our rivers, lakes, and streams for the contamination of much of the food we eat and even the water we drink. While half the world's scientists and engineers are employed to produce the technological weaponry of modern war, some thirty-five percent of humanity has no access to safe drinking water. Our unbridled craving for domination has made us our own worst enemies. The ultimate medical nemesis is to be found within ourselves and the institutions which express our values. For health education to succeed we need to address ourselves to the things which truly make us unhealthy; we need to redefine our relationship to the Earth and to each other. This is the point at which health education and moral education coalesce.

It is in this chapter of the book that we provide a heuristic alternative to the traditional way in which our culture has conceptualized its relationship with nature. Drawing together a panoply of developments from different fields, we show that a science of discovery is possible in which the driving value is not power and domination over nature, but *participation and connection.* Recognizing that human consciousness cannot be isolated and extracted from the things of which it is conscious, we postulate a wholistic epistemology in which knowing is directed towards integration rather than division, participation with nature rather than separation from it.

The goal of health for all will not become reality unless the theory which motivates it is sufficiently free of scientism to appreciate that wholism is an integral part of the philosophy of health, allowing for personal and societal needs to be realized in a global context.

CHAPTER 1

The epistemological evolution of reductionist medical science

The link forged between medicine and science is an ancient and venerable one, though the science of the ancients could hardly be equated with the formal science of today. While there is considerable debate over the birth, legitimate or otherwise, of formal science, [1] it is clear that medicine has predominately relied upon the prevailing views of its times well before science as we know it was the view that prevailed. As Singer and Underwood have put it, "Scientific medicine began with the Greeks. But, just as there were brave men before Agamemnon, so there were men who practiced the art of healing long before the time of the Greek physicians."[2, 3] Practitioners of enormously different intellectual habits have, since prehistoric times, been engaged in the healing of the sick. Research findings drawn from physical anthropology, in combination with paleopathology (the study of fossil and other manifestations of disease in prehistoric humans) and paleodemography (the study of vital statistics including disease manifestations of ancient populations); have in recent years provided an important source of literature on the origins, patterns, and forms of ancient medicine. Tests using X-rays and microscopic examination of ancient fossils have revealed that disease was coincident with the first forms of life on this planet. Similar studies have shown that at least 25,000 years before the Christian era, humans were plagued with diseases such as rachitism, osteitis, and acromegaly.[4] The remains of Egyptian mummies exhibit pleuritic and arteriosclerotic lesions. Prehistoric fossils reveal not only information about ancient disease states but also about ancient healing practices. Remains of ancient skulls have revealed evidence, for example, of early healing practice in the form of trephination holes. Within the context of modern surgical procedures, a trephination hole is an opening drilled through the skull to the brain in the hope of mitigating the build-up of abnormal pressures normally resulting from head injuries. An intriguing difference between the modern and the ancient use of trephination, however, lies in the fact that ancient skulls with trephine holes do not in general betray signs of cranial injury. This being so, paleopathologists have inferred that the ancients employed trephination for magical or supernatural purposes, with the intention, say, of exorcising demons of evil spirits, thereby remedying the disease states and other afflictions of the body which were presumed to accompany them. Other evidence gathered from a wide variety of sources, including the analysis of bone and fossil specimens, has given rise to the hypothesis that prehistoric humans made use of massage, herbalist treatments, poultices, bone-setting, and even dieting. [5,6]

The origins of medicine in magic and religion

There is little doubt that the early shamans, witch doctors, and priests appealed to the realm of the supernatural and magic to explain and control sundry natural phenomena whose patterns augured the good or ill health of whole tribes or of specific individuals within them. In an attempt to manipulate the forces of nature, some of which all too frequently wreaked havoc upon them, the ancients incorporated the original 'science' of healing as a component of their supernatural or religious belief system. Common events such as famine and plague were thereby understood and responded to in a context of interpretation in which the world was populated by spirit forces and unmasterable demons. Endeavoring to make these impersonal forces more comprehensible and thus more tractable, the ancients transformed the world of impersonal spirits conceptually into a world of personal gods, possessed of some of the same attributes as the human, and in some cases animal creatures over which they were deemed to rule. While the savage force of the wind was without ears, for instance, it was at least possible to implore the god of tempests to calm the angry sea. It was at least possible, that is to say, to supplicate the gods or appease them if need be, and homage and sacrifice came to feature as the accepted modes of petition. Within this framework of belief, sickness and health depended primarily upon the caprice of the gods, their sense of justice, and their willingness to be entreated by their human subjects. Out of primitive religion came a primitive science of adaptation, and medicine became even more culturally intertwined with religious belief. Although polytheism gave way eventually to monotheism, the symbiosis between medicine and religion was preserved. Living in accordance with God's law in ancient times not frequently determinative of the "law of the land," came to function along with humble entreaty as the way in which religion shaped the cultural milieu in respect of which the health problems of the times were defined and treated.

Whether an individual had violated social or religious taboos, or even had nightmares, began to figure in the conceptual scheme in which disease and its prognosis could be religiously understood. Biological functions and malfunctions of the living organism were often construed in supernatural terms. In many cultures it was believed that disease was the punishment which the gods inflicted upon those who dared to sin or rebel against them. Even the bodily intrusion of evil spirits and devils was sometimes explained by reference to the violations of taboos or a straying from belief, thereby incurring the loss of protection (personal immunity) otherwise provided by the gods. Unsurprisingly, the medical relevance of personal hygiene was covertly and overtly enshrined in religious prohibitions forbidding the consumption of certain foods or legislating for their special preparation. Oblations prior to eating, along with incantations or prayers in relation to the planting, harvesting, and consumption of food, were similarly ritualized.[7,8]

What might at first glance be regarded as an obscure relation between religion and medicine reveals a profound insight into the character of human well-being. Within religious tradition of various persuasions there has often been a persistent emphasis upon the subtle interface between "well-being" and "doing-good", and thus indirectly upon the interplay between health and virtue.[9] Each dimension of human need, be it physical, mental, or spiritual, was characterized as having a realm of proper expression. Although the delicate equilibrium between the needs of the flesh and the needs of the spirit has not always been preserved in practice within some religious traditions, the basic perception of the contribution to health through commitment to the "good life" or the "moral code" has throughout the ages figured as an intrinsic feature of the religious orientation.

The history of the relation between medicine and religion has, in different places and in different times, been decidedly ambiguous, and while there is no uniform logical progression away from religion to science, the transition of medicine to the reductionist-mechanist paradigm can be coherently discerned. By the time of the early Egyptian and Babylonian civilizations, for example, a partial schism between medicine and religion had already begun to appear. Having come to be recognized as the technicians of medicine, the herbalists affirmed a naturalist philosophy of medicine which inadvertently alienated the shamans and priests with whom the more mystical functions of ancient religious medicine, including poultices, exorcism, and the reading of spiritual omens, remained. The historical stage was thus set, albeit in an inchoate way, for the eventual division of labor which would culminate in opposing schools of thought.[10,11]

The philosophical disparity between the Vitalist and Mechanist schools affords one conspicuous example of the conceptual shift of medicine from its basis in religious thought to its new home in reductionist science. Resolved to articulate a non-materialist interpretation of living organisms, the Vitalists, for example, held firmly to the idea that while the living body is composed of inanimate parts, there is an entity or "life-force" not reducible to those parts and in virtue of which those same inanimate parts function as the parts of a living organism. George Ernst Stahl (1660-1734), who popularized the Vitalist view, believed that the word "machine" expressed what the body was not. To Stahl living matter was not governed by physical and chemical laws as was non-living matter but rather by a sensitive soul. Aristotle's treatises On the Soul and On the Generation of Animals have been influential in determining subsequent developments within the Vitalist school.[12,13] This identification of the biological life of an organism with its psyche, for example, inspired a theory and practice of medicine in which the biological activities of the parts of a living organism were to be understood by reference to the organizational form of the whole which enshrined an aspect of a more comprehensive "life-force" independent of it. Chemical and physical processes were, to the Vitalists, slaves of the sensitive soul, and in attempting to understand these processes Vitalism inadvertently gave rise to the eighteenth-century study of physiology. For it was in this century, with the mathematical explanations of Isaac Newton, that biologists sought to order their knowledge through the application of philosophical principles, and Vitalism was one approach.

In their defection from the religious metaphysics associated with Vitalism, the Mechanists sought material explanation for disease. Increasingly preoccupied with the analysis of disease rather than health, the Mechanists inspired a radical change in the orientation of health care. With health being defined by them exclusively as the absence of disease and disease as a breakdown or malfunction in the mechanical parts of the biological organism, the concept of disease as a disorder of the whole person diminished in importance. The physician or practitioner's attention was thus diverted from 'whole-person' treatment to 'person-part' treatment. Resolutely affirming the machinelike character of the human organism, mechanist medicine fostered an interventionist orientation in which repair of the body required the expertise of a trained body mechanic.

The difference of philosophical disposition signified by the Vitalist and Mechanist schools gave rise to a conceptual cleavage within medicine which has contributed significantly to our present medical heritage. Given the complex sociocultural entwinement of the craft of healing with magic, religion, and philosophy, the institutional dominance of conventional medical science took nearly two thousand years, the influence of religious philosophy dominating one cultural epoch, the influence of science progressively dominating the other.

Greek, Roman and Arab traditions in healing

Hippocrates of Cos and his followers could with justification be applauded as the forerunners not only of the mechanistic tradition within medicine, but of the causal theory of medicine as well. In one of the treatises attributed to Hippocrates, titled, the "Sacred Disease of Epilepsy," is described as not being "any more divine or sacred than any other disease but, on the contrary, [as having] specific characteristics and a definite cause." [14, 15, 16, 17]

The philosophical influences which shaped the causal-mechanist tradition of Hippocratic medicine are exceedingly diverse and convoluted. The Hippocratic School reflected an uneasy amalgam of disparate world-views, rituals, and philosophical beliefs which came over the centuries to be synthesized as a consequence of vicissitudes of trade, political or religious domination, and even military conquest.

From the Minoan civilization dating back to the eleventh century BC derived an awareness of the importance of hygiene, though Minoan hygiene was then mingled with temple medicine and serpent cults. Eventually, the interest in hygiene would in Hellenic times be reflected in the worship of Hygeia, one of the most significant of the early healing deities. A manifestation of the Cretan goddess Athena, the Minoan symbolism of the snake and mistletoe panacea was preserved despite three waves of barbarian invasions into Greece by the end of the second millennium BC. As a result of the barbarian imposition of patriarchal religion, Hygeia was reconceptualized as the daughter of the male god Asclepius whose name is etymologically associated with the ancient Greek word for mistletoe. Hygeia's snakes survived the assimilation by coiling around the staff of Asclepius, the origin of the Caduceus, which has of course bequeathed itself as the symbol of western medicine. [18]

In the sixth century BC, Ionian philosophy carried forward the Minoan legacy, adding to it the astrology, demonology, and the materia medica (the use of chemical substances for healing) of Mesopotamian culture. This was supplemented by the advances of Egyptian physicians in pharmacopeia, surgical procedures, and their own deification, giving a whole new sense to the "doctor's word as law." [19] Often acclaimed as the first human medical figure in history, Imhotep, the famed Egyptian healer was subsequently deified by the Greeks and equated with Asclepius. Although the Ionian medical schools of Cos and Crides provided a rich source from which Hippocratic medicine of the fifth and fourth centuries BC would take its general medical inheritance, it was the Aristotelian views of the fourth century that supplied the specific philosophical foundation of Hippocratic medicine. While Aristotelian philosophy of medicine had incorporated the Sicilian reliance upon pheumatism and dissection, it also adopted and refined the concept of material causality as the basis for understanding the symptoms and signs of disease and their origins. Even the so-called "sacred diseases" such as epilepsy were reconceptualized by Hippocrates as natural afflictions. On Hippocrates's view there were - contrary to the conventional wisdom of his day - many different types of disease, not just one single disease. Coupled with the Aristotelian notion of material causality, the concept of a plurality of diseases set the framework in which the search for specific causes of specific diseases could be initiated. [20, 21]

Although Hippocrates himself was determined that medicine should be practiced as a discipline rather than Aristotelian natural science, he displayed in his writings, particularly in Airs, Waters, and Places, a keen awareness of a variety of environmental factors influencing health. Cognizant of the fundamental interdependence of body and mind, and the influence of the environment upon both, his famous theory that any quantitative impairment in the balance of the body's four humors (blood, yellow bile, black bile, and phlegm) would produce disease betrayed his wholistic approach to medicine even through this expression of his commitment to the causal theory of disease. [22, 23] The role of the physician was not to intervene directly to re-establish the balance among the humors, but to strengthen the natural healing powers of the body, vis medicatrix naturae, to make whatever adjustments were required. His stress upon lifestyle, including the role in health maintenance played by fresh food and water, air quality, even the topography of the land and climate, laid the foundations for an integrative theory of medicine which would shortly be abandoned by those who followed him.

When the seat of Hellenic learning was transferred from Athens to Alexandria where the first university in the world had just been founded, along with what would become one of the most famous libraries in history, the causal aspects of Hippocrates's medical philosophy were hypostasized and given a priority in the Alexandrian theory of medicine which they had not previously enjoyed. Attracting learned practitioners of medicine from around the ancient world, the citadel of Alexandria boasted of scholars such as Archimedes, Eratosthenes, Strabo, and Euclid, whose thought would inspire a progressively mechanistic and reductionist theory of medicine. The Alexandrian school was celebrated for its contribution to the science of anatomical dissection and surgery, largely under the direction of Herophilius of Chalcedon (335-280), the father of anatomy, and Erasistratus (c. 310-250), famed for his surgical exploits and the discovery of the tricuspid valve. [24, 25] With this almost exclusive focus upon the material causes of disease and the physician's direct intervention to extirpate them, Hippocrates's appreciation of the complex interplay between disease, its genesis in the disruption of the internal harmony of the body, and environmental factors affecting that harmony was gradually dissipated in favor of a far more restricted and interventionist view of the locus of disease in specific organs and parts of the human body. Given the conviction that only natural rather than supernatural forces could be enlisted to explain disease and the treatment relevant to it, the causal mechanics of medicine ensured that Vitalism was suppressed. Inasmuch as the proceedings of the gods, the power of prayer and the life of values associated with religious belief were deemed to be extraneous to the new science of medicine, the notion that disease should be seen as a disorder of the whole person systematically diminished. In the end Hippocrates's wholistic orientation towards medicine was distorted to reflect only one aspect of it, and the resultant preoccupation with biological explanations for disease inspired a reductionist-mechanist paradigm which would come to dominate the theory and practice of medicine.

The Romans borrowed their orientation to medicine largely from the Greeks. Priests of the cult of Asclepius appear to have been the first major practitioners of medicine, followed by slaves, and then freed slaves, until Gaius Julius Caesar's edict in 46 BC that Roman citizenship would be granted to all freeborn Greek physicians practicing in Rome. Indeed, it is alleged that the first Greek physicians to have practiced in Rome was Archagathus (c. 220 BC), a surgeon and also a freed slave. It was under the tutelage of Asclepiades of Bithyria (mid-first century) and the sophisticated Celsus (early first century) that the standard of medicine and medical training in Rome improved. Celsus's compilation of the medical learning of this time, De re medica, written about 30

AD, is reputed to be the first classical medical text to have been printed (c. 1478). It was Celsus who also defined the first four of the cardinal signs of inflammation: pain (dolor), redness (rubor), heat (calor) and swelling (tumor); the fifth sign, loss of function, was added a century later. [26, 27] In the early second century AD, treatises on midwifery and gynecology were written by Coranus Ephesus. The anatomical orientation was strong and organs and parts of the body purported to be diseased were treated with drugs or simply removed, most often with disastrous results for the patient, by primitive surgery. In those days' students of medicine practiced vivisection on criminals and comparative anatomy on apes. Although a number of schools (e.g., the Methodist, the Pneumatic, and the Eclectic) flourished in Rome throughout the first and second centuries AD, the causal-mechanist position had gained a strong philosophical foothold, and the subtlety of Hippocrates's wholistic approach was lost almost altogether.[28]

It was around the second century that the advent of Galenic medicine provided a further impetus to the causal-mechanist model. The vast writings of Galen were on the one hand philosophical and on the other hand descriptive, and some of his works contain an uneasy amalgam of both philosophical and descriptive elements. Occupying a virtually unique position of pre-eminence among the medical scientists of his time, he espoused in his protracted treatise *Peri Apodexixeos* ("On Demonstration") a theory of scientific knowledge which relied upon and amplified the causal-mechanistic paradigm contained in Aristotle's *Posterior Analytics.* Also influenced by Hippocrates, on whose work he wrote fifteen commentaries, Galen recast the Hippocratic doctrine of the humors, arguing that the body consisted of anatomical parts (not humors) which provide the true causal explanation of disease. Galen enunciated principles of anatomy which have served as the authoritative basis of the subject even in recent centuries. It was Galen, for example, who determined that the arteries carried blood. [29, 30]

Impressed by Hippocrates's account of *physis,* i.e., the natural healing powers of the body, Galen was a firm advocate of personal hygiene as a form of preventive medicine, and did much to promote the cause of sanitary engineering in Rome. In this regard Galen's support for and encouragement of the Roman's interest in collective hygiene, the effective provision of drinking water, gymnasiums, and public baths, did much to promote the progress of community health and the eradication of disease in ways only partially indicated by the mechanistic orientation of his philosophy. While the teleological tenor of his theory of physiology was never, altogether, reconciled with his causal-mechanistic theory of anatomy, his view of the nature of the human body contained a presumption in favor of causal mechanics which subsumed his teleology and the wholism that might have derived from it. Galen did not - despite his prolific writings - establish formally a teaching school of medicine, and upon his death (c. 200), the substantial medical knowledge he accrued was for a while lost in what has been called the "Dark Ages of Medicine."

With the collapse of the western half of the Roman Empire in the fifth century, the ongoing process of the consolidation of medicine on the basis of a distinct corpus of philosophical assumptions about the nature of the human body, in conjunction with the medical theory which followed from it and the public health practices to which it led, were all badly disrupted. Throughout the Middle Ages, the sinuosities of the evolution of medicine made its history more difficult to trace and the expression of its philosophical underpinning less coherent. Under the protection of the great *basileis*, the rulers of the Byzantine Empire, the eastern part of the Roman Empire and its capital of Constantinople became the axis of the Christian world until it was conquered by the Turks in the fifteenth century, when the Ottoman Empire was established. [31] Byzantine medicine until that time vacillated between the scholarly pursuit of past medical learning on the one hand and the Christian orthodox interpretation of disease and illness on the other. Medical scholarship and the philosophy of causal-mechanist medicine was preserved by compilers such as Aitios (c.500), Alexander of Tralles (mid-sixth century), and Paul of Aegina (c. 625-690). On the other hand, the rigid Christian orthodoxy of the Eastern Empire reinstated a conservative view of the religious nature of disease and illness. Those afflicted with illness were reckoned as potential saints. Heresy was specifically regarded as disease, and a whole host of degenerative conditions of the body were equated with its signs. God was reaffirmed as the supreme healer, the priest as his consort in healing. [32]

With the collapse of the Western Empire the Middle Ages witnessed not only the birth of feudalism but a stellar ascendancy of the Church Fathers, who saw themselves as the guardians of all knowledge. Although lamentable, their part in the destruction of the Library of Alexandria, with its immense accumulation of medical learning, simply on the ground that it was pagan, was hardly surprising. As in the Byzantine tradition, healing figured predominately as the prerogative of the Church, and disease was once again reconceived as the punishment for sin and apostasy. Sickness was a sign of alienation from God. Acting on God's behalf, the priest offered salvation as the universal panacea and the Church as his residential hospital. The cure for disease was repentance and self-flagellation. Dissection of the human body was, except in exceptional circumstances, regarded as desecration, and anatomical investigations into its intricate workings were frowned upon. Living in constant fear of God and confronted by a social reality of plagues, pestilence, fires, floods, drought, and famine, the general populace found the lure of some of the more "unholy" forms of healing difficult to resist. [33, 34] Despite its persistent efforts to discourage medical alternatives to Christian orthodoxy, the Church's parochial position on illness and disease actually contributed to the proliferation of cults professing the curative or healing powers of witchcraft, magic, astrology, amulets, relics, and even elves and fairies.

The scientific medicine of the Hellenic tradition and the causal theory of disease underpinning it survived the fall of Rome in the hands of the great Arab physicians of the Middle East, Jundi Shapur, the birthplace of Moorish medicine, was built on the Persian desert by Nestorius in the fifth century upon his exile from Constantinople on a charge of heresy. Within a few centuries the Eastern Caliphate had achieved a reputation of medical distinction, due largely to its array of illustrious physicians such as al-Tabari (838-923), Rhazes (865-925), Haly Abbas (930-994), and Avicenna (980-1037), all of whom in various ways affirmed a fundamental connection between disease and material causes of a biological kind. With a predilection for alchemy, Moorish medicine concentrated on the chemical analysis of living matter, with the aim of showing that disease could be explicated biochemically. In Avicenna's *Canon Medicinae,* one of the most popular works in the history of medicine, the author was concerned to assimilate and synthesize the medical philosophies of Aristotle and Galen in the service of a reductionist biology of medicine. Avicenna's emphasis on the chemical origins of disease laid the conceptual foundations for the inception of modern bio-chemistry and gave medicine a reductionist orientation in respect of which a separate discipline (i.e., biochemistry) could be brought to bear on its subject-matter. [35, 36] The Hellenistic conceptual inheritance was thus used by the Arabs to establish a methodological framework in which medical understanding was made increasingly dependent upon the technological capacity required to affect the analysis of the complex structure of the human body in terms of a malfunction within its constituent parts.

Fanatically inspired by the teachings of Mohammed, the sphere of Arab dominance soon extended from Cathay to Spain, thereby eroding the Church's aegis of power and control over medical learning. The reductionist approach to medicine was thus promulgated in the Western Caliphate by physicians of Moorish medicine such as the surgeon Abul Kasim (c. 936-1013), Avenzoar the clinician (c. 1091-1162), the philosopher-surgeon Averroes (1126-1198), and Maimonides, the Jewish humanist and private physician to the sultan Saladin. [37] Among the other contributions made by Arabs to western medicine, one of the most significant from the vantage of promoting a reductionist philosophy of medicine was the organization of pharmacy and the standardization of specific drugs for specific ailments. The study of pharmacology became of such huge proportion that it became necessary to separate the profession of doctor from that of the chemist. [38]

During the period of the Crusades monasteries became the institutional vehicles for the expression of religious medicine, which by this time had been strongly influenced by the causal theory of disease and illness and by the Arab reliance upon reductionist biochemistry for its eradication. Having located their sites in propinquity to the arduous routes traveled by pilgrims, monasteries naturally functioned as places of refuge and recovery from the toil of journey. Pilgrims sought from monasteries not only worship, respite, and news, but also healing. Given the traditional function of monasteries as places of religious study, their involvement in aiding sick or injured pilgrims led inevitably to a concern for additional medical training and knowledge. Monte Cassino, for example, founded in the sixth century, was the monastery where the monk Constantine, the African, translated various Arabic readings of classical Greek medicine into Latin at the close of the first millennium. A century later in Toledo, scholars of Christian, Jewish, and Arab persuasion displayed unprecedented religious tolerance by collaborating in the translation of classical medical treatises from Syrian and Arabic into Latin. As monasteries diversified their activities towards scholarship on the one hand and the provision of medical care on the other, they inadvertently helped to set up the institutional context in which the establishment of formal universities and hospitals could follow. One of the most famous centers of medicine in the Middles Ages was the School of Salerno. Originating as a pilgrim hospital attached to a Benedictine monastery, the Salernian School separated medicine from the control of the priests and made available places for men and women of all countries to study. This school enjoyed a good reputation well into the thirteenth century, but with the establishment of bigger schools it gradually diminished in importance, though did not cease to exist until 1811 following a decree of suppression issued by Napoleon I. [39]

By the twelfth century universities were founded at Bologna, Padua, Montpellier, Paris, and later at Oxford and Cambridge, though medical teaching was at first entirely theoretical with little or no clinical instruction. Bologna had an organized medical faculty as early as 1156, from whence came a strong anatomical and surgical tradition, highly dependent upon Galen's earlier causal-mechanistic paradigm. It was Henri de Mondeville (1260-1325), a student of Bologna, who ensured that the mechanist model was adopted by French physicians when he returned to and settled at the famous Montpellier medical school. [40] Mundinus (1275-1326), one of Mondeville's contemporaries who became known as the "Restorer of Anatomy," did much to advance the notion that material explanations for disease could be enunciated in anatomical terms. Unlike the professors who succeeded him, Mundinus dissected personally, teaching his students by practical example. Reading from textbooks, his successors were not to sit exaltedly in a high chair, watching as a demonstrator prosecuted the body under the guidance of an ostensor. The students, in emulation of the professor, wore academic dress and did not personally take part. [41] Among Padua's distinguished physicians was the famed Polish astronomer Nicholas Copernicus (1473-1543), whose mechanist philosophy of science also permeated his approach to medicine.

It was not, however, until the Renaissance that the next stage in the evolution of reductio-mechanist medicine took place. Paralleling Renaissance excitement about the discovery and exploration of new places and continents was a fervent desire to explore anatomically the human body itself. With the invention of the printing press the records and distribution of medical scholarship, particularly anatomical diagrams, was facilitated. It was in this social milieu of a new appreciation of interest in the human body that Michelangelo, Leonardo da Vinci, and other artists pursued dissection as a means of securing the knowledge required to represent more accurately the human body in its finest detail. About the time da Vinci died in 1518, a child named Vesalius was also showing a keen interest in the anatomical structure of the body. Much of academic anatomy at the time was based on the treatises of Galen, and Vesalius was determined to test Galen's submissions on these matters firsthand. His celebrated tome *De Humani Corporis Fabrica,* published in 1543, contained countless case studies of anatomical investigations, the synthesis of which provided new methodological principles of analysis, and contributed significantly to the scientific tradition of Padua which stressed the importance of living anatomy (i.e., the study of the minute anatomical mechanisms of the body in action or of the nature of the structures governing their potential action). [42,43]

Combined with the Renaissance craving for learning in general was a specific philosophy which dictated how things should be learnt. Although the application of this philosophy differed among the scholars and scientists of the time, its pervasive influence shaped the notion that the best and perhaps the only way of truly comprehending the deepest secrets of nature lay in reducing the complex of nature to the fundamental parts of which it is composed. One of the great rebels of the Renaissance was Philippus Aureolus Paracelsus (c. 1493-1541) who spent much of his lifetime as an itinerant physician. Paracelsus became a legend in his own time as an iconoclast when he attacked the works of Galen and Avicenna on the grounds of dogmatism and made a public bonfire in the city center of Basel out of their writings. [44,45] Notwithstanding his animosity towards their work, he affirmed his own commitment to the causal theory of disease, which they shared, postulating that diseases were actual entities for which remedies could be found in nature. His belief in the curative powers of minerals, tinctures, and essences thus reinforced the inchoate and emergent tradition of medicinal chemistry.

The birth of medical science and the concept of the body as machine

A more decisive impetus to the reductio-mechanist tradition in medicine, however, was provided by Galileo (1564-1642), for it was he who combined mathematics with scientific experimentation to deduce the mechanistic laws which he believed governed the behavior of all phenomena. Reputed to be the first thinker to explore systematically the relation between mathematics and empirical experimentation, he has come to be known as the father of modern science. His distinction between the essential and nonessential properties of matter was of monumental importance in advancing the reductionist paradigm. [46, 47] The essential properties of material bodies signified their quantifiable aspects, e.g., weight, shape, height, movement, etc. Non-essential properties referred to those aspects of bodies such as taste, smell, sound, color, etc., which were presumed to reflect the 'subjective' rather than the 'objective' components of the subject-matter of science. The possibility of the mathematical analysis of nature and all that it contains, Galileo averred, depends upon restricting the scope of science and its investigations to the measurable or "primary" properties of matter, thereby excluding the non-quantifiable, "secondary" ones. [48] In short, the domain of subjective experience, feelings, motives, intentions, the qualitative or value aspects of human experience are deliberately eschewed by Galilean science.

While it is clear that the philosophical underpinnings of Galileo's new science were decidedly mechanist, it is not simply the reductio-mechanistic methodology which inhibits the development of medical knowledge; it is that to which nature has been reduced. The objective language of nature was cast as mathematics, and the secrets of nature revealed mathematically. The ultimate character and structure of nature is revealed by reducing it to the basic mathematical or geometrical relations of which it is constituted. In the context of medicine, the reduction ensures that the subjective self or personhood has, by implication, been divorced from the quantifiable aspects of its embodiment. The impact of Galileo's thought on the evolution of medicine has thus been momentous. It was Santorio Santorio (1561-1636) who first applied the Galilean principles of measurement to biological matters, inventing firstly the *pulsilogium* with which the pulse rate could be measured and later adapting the Galilean thermometer to measure the body temperature. [49]

Francis Bacon (1560-1626) in the second book of his work *Of the Advancement of Learning,* however, warned of the trend to reduce mankind to parts when he wrote: "So we see also that the science of medicine if it be destitute and forsaken by natural philosophy, it is not much better than an empirical practice."[50] Bacon was well aware of the significance of the emotions and the class interaction between the mind and the body. "For the lineaments of the body do disclose the disposition and inclination of the mind in general; but the motions of the countenance and parts do not only so; but do further disclose the present humor and state of the mind as well."[51]

Contemporary with Galileo and Bacon was the distinguished philosopher Rene Descartes (1596-1650) whose philosophy of science closely paralleled that of Galileo. Not unlike Galileo, Descartes perceived the true structure of nature as reducible to mathematical relations describing its most fundamental constituents. According to Descartes, however, the material world was no more than a machine. Just as the workings of a watch could be explained in terms of the relation of its parts, so too the material world admitted of explanation through the analysis of its parts, their arrangement, and their interaction. The method Descartes employed in this reduction was the analytic method, and it has since come to figure paradigmatically as the instrument of reductionism in medicine and in epistemology. The concept of analysis and the concept of reduction have important similarities, though they need not be coterminous in extension. Analysis is in essence the method of divide-and-conquer. Analysis amounts to epistemic reductionism only when it is crystallized into a dogma holding that the complexity of nature, and all that it contains, can be exhaustively known and explained by way of its analysis. On this reading the reductionist theory of knowledge becomes obstinately analytic, delimiting *a priori* the framework of scientific investigation in reductionist terms. Once this point is clear, it is easier to appreciate that bioreductionism in medicine is simply one discipline-oriented expression of the reductionist theory of knowledge in general. Although it may not have been Descartes' intention that analysis should be used in this reductionist manner, there is no doubt that it has been so used. The philosophical search for the foundations of knowledge within science has been paralleled with medicine by the search for the foundations or fundamental properties of life.

To appreciate the full impact of Descartes' thought upon science and medicine, however, it is imperative to couple his concept of analysis with his doctrine of dualism. Descartes' partition between mind and matter represented a fundamental distinction between two distinct realms, but it was the separation of *res cognitans* from *res extensa* that made it possible for the first time to describe the word of res extensa as a machine whose workings could be reduced to mechanical laws. It was only by following Galileo's lead of separating the quantifiable from the non-quantifiable that matter could be characterized in purely mechanical terms without reference to non-quantifiable properties. Descartes' way of achieving this was to extract from matter the non-quantifiable property of mind and spirit. Descartes did however believe that the mind and body could interact, as Hall suggests: "This system was, for Descartes, an *extended entity,* a corpuscular mechanism arranged to act, in most of our behaviors, reflexively or independently of the *cogitant entity,* mind - but also able to interact with mind when circumstances required." [52] The ramifications of Descartes' division were far-reaching, transforming not only the philosophical foundation of science and paving the way for the development of Newtonian mechanics, but also profoundly altering the attitude taken by science to the human body, its multifarious functions reducing to mechanical operations. Some proponents of the reductionist-mechanist model, such as Julien Offray De La Mettrie and the Iatro-mechanists who preceded him, went so far as to assert that the human body did not simply behave like a machine, but actually was a machine. The theory of medicine and the practice of medicine which followed from it were also altered accordingly. As Fritjof Capra has put it:

> The Cartesian division between mind and matter has had a profound effect on Western thought. It has taught us to be aware of ourselves as isolated egos existing "inside" our bodies; it has led us to set a higher value on mental manual work; it has enabled huge industries to sell products—especially to women—that would make us owners of the "ideal body"; it has kept doctors from seriously considering the psychological dimensions of illness and psychotherapists from dealing with their patients' bodies. [53]

The transition from the Cartesian to the Newtonian picture of the world is unencumbered. It was Newton, not Descartes, who provided the systematic mathematical articulation of Descartes' mechanistic vision of nature, though Gattfried Leibniz (1646-1716), philosopher, scientist, and mathematician, has also been credited with the intervention of calculus. Whether it was Newton or Leibniz to whom the development of the differential calculus can be attributed, it is clear that calculus afforded a system of mathematical description more sophisticated and comprehensive than any previous mathematical scheme. Newtonian mechanics set the stage not only for the future development of the medical sciences for the next three centuries but for the particular direction that development would take. The degree of development within the medical sciences thus came to be judged proportionally to the degree of formalized reduction secured within them. Medical understanding of the nature of the human body and its workings was reckoned to be a matter of the progressive revelation of the structure of its fundamental parts. The historical progression led medical science to analyze the body in terms first of its appendages, then its internal organs, and later to the cells of which those organs are constituted, and more recently, to the genetic components of which the cells are made, DNA, the ultimate building-blocks, we are told, of all living organisms. Newtonian mechanics thus provided the conceptual categories required to consolidate the various forms of reductionist disposition into a coherent framework of scientific understanding which would in due course profoundly influence the whole scientific approach. Incorporating the Galilean and Cartesian stress upon a reductionist mechanics, the Hellenic commitment to the causal theory of disease was reinstated as a science of *quantitative* analysis. Inasmuch as quantitative analysis favored a science of mensuration (measurement analysis); the reductionist program claimed for itself an objectivity within medicine which could itself be measured.

In the seventeenth century anatomical progress within the reductionist model was impressive. Robert Boyle (1627-1691), known as the Father of Chemistry, demonstrated that air is a material substance and necessary to support respiration. Robert Hook (1635-1703), an assistant of Boyle's, went on to publish in 1665 *Micrographia*, the first text showing microscopic objects and introducing for the first time the notion of a "cell" or compartment in plant and animals. [54, 55] The shift from the study of external parts of the body to a study of its internal organs was facilitated by Wirsung's isolation of the pancreatic duct, by Glisson's analysis of the liver, by Stenson's work on the parotid gland, and van Leuwenhoek's ophthalmological discoveries. But the truly outstanding medical scientist of the seventeenth century was William Harvey (1568-1657), who studied in Cambridge and in Padua, where the influence upon him of Fabricius ab Acquapendente (1533-1619) would be indelible. We have in this chapter already commented upon Galilean reductionism, Newtonian mechanism, and their impact upon the scientific world. What we have not remarked upon, and this aspect of Galileo's thinking was equally important for Harvey, was Galileo's exposition of the concept of *motion* as a vehicle for explaining the varying relations among heavenly bodies. For it was motion that would serve as a catalyst in the formulation of Harvey's account of the body as a *machine* in which blood was moved by the heart in a systematic cycle through the body. The movement or circulation of blood was believed to be measurable, as were the specific factors which might serve to inhibit its cycle. The very great debt which modern physiology owes to Harvey is undeniable to anyone who opens a contemporary book on physiology.

The development of the microscope both betrayed and reinforced the seventeenth century disposition to explain the workings of the human body as a machine by decomposing it to its smallest parts. Although the microscope is presumed to have been invented c. 1590 by Janssen, it was Antonius Van Leeuwenhoek (1632-1723), a cloth merchant from Delft and spare-time glass grinder, who perfected it and described what was later to be confirmed by Marcello Malpighi (1628-1694), the capillary blood circulation. Malpighi went on to pioneer microscopic anatomy, extending and refining Harvey's theory of circulation. [56] The microscope assisted also in the confirmation of lymphatic circulation, supposedly first observed by Aselli (1581-1626) and later corroborated by Riolan (1577-1657) and Pecquet (1622-1674). By demonstrating - contrary to the conventional wisdom of the time - that lymph does not enter the liver but rather circulates through special vessels, their work challenged the role of central importance given to the liver in the Galenic system and thus paved the way conceptually for the implementation of a coherent reductionist theory of anatomy. [57] The earlier architectonic anatomical theories of Vesalius (1541-1564) were in a sense finally realized in the discovery that the body contained not one but two principal fluids of circulation, blood and lymph.

With the advent of Newtonian mechanics the conceptual path for the defection of medicine from religion to science was thus virtually complete. Europe of the eighteenth century, however, was yet to bear witness to the bitter struggle between Church and State as the institution of science gained sufficient political momentum to supplant the established institution of religion. The laws of religion, once completely dominant within academies and universities, were rapidly being replaced by the laws of science. The proliferation of scientific journals augmented not only the social status but the mystique of science. The mystique of science was further enhanced by its employment of a technical vocabulary, thus creating the impression of erudition and the creation of a language all its own. Although Cotton Mather (1663-1728) was both a pastor and a physician, it was the scientific and not the religious thrust of his battle against smallpox, in the specific form of inoculations that brought him fame. By promoting the scientific eradication of one of the most deadly and virulent strains of disease, Mather had in the services of mankind unwittingly struck a blow for the authority of reductionist-mechanist science against religion. [58] The technological success of science clearly enhanced its authority. The enunciation by Euler and Watt of other mechanist principles of physics, some of which in turn led, for example, to the discovery of the new force of electricity, did much to revolutionize the world. A confirmation of the power of reductionism, electricity served to increase popular support and create a social reverence for science. Along with popular support came financial support for governments, communities, organizations, and individual benefactors. Science was now able to compete with religion in financial terms, and with virtually every scientific breakthrough, it found itself competing successfully for all the financial resources society could muster

Financial support for the new science of medicine encouraged revolutionary changes in medical teaching, with the establishment of new medical schools such as the Old Vienna School, founded by Gerard van Swieten (1700-1772), and the renewal of others such as the Edinburgh School where William Heberden (1710-1801) wrote the first classic description of angina pectoris (severe paroxysmal pain in the chest). Giovanni Morgagni (1682-1771), appointed Professor of Anatomy at Padua in 1715, linked for the first time the anatomical concept to the practice of medicine. By distinguishing between normal and abnormal pathological anatomy, he correlated gross lesions and symptoms. [59, 60] Dramatic changes in clinical teaching were introduced by Hermann Boerhave (1668-1738) who, as Professor of Clinical Medicine at Leiden, carried out the teaching of medicine to more than half the physicians of Europe in a small teaching hospital. While the eighteenth century was a period of intense political and religious struggles, the reductionist tradition in medical science continued to advance.

Universities and academies featured as the centers of intellectual life, and a plethora of journals came into existence, thereby facilitating the proliferation of reductionist experiments and approaches to research. Progress in the natural sciences was no less than spectacular and the success enjoyed in the natural sciences filtered through to the medical science parasitic upon them. Antoine Laurent Lavoisier (1743-1794) and Joseph Priestly (1733-1804) made the discovery of oxygen independently of each other. The physiology of respiration initiated by Robert Boyle (1627-1691) was refined by Lavoisier who elaborated the analogy between combustion and homeostasis. Before eventually suffering death at the blade of the guillotine he managed to prove that the absorption of oxygen, along with the combustion of hydrogen and carbon, duplicated the essential process of respiration. The "father of modern chemistry" had thus demonstrated unequivocally that the biological functions of living organisms depend upon chemical processes. The titan of physiology during this period, however, was Albrecht von Haller (1708-1777), of Swiss nationality. Von Haller, author of some two thousand scientific articles, and another fourteen thousand letters on subjects ranging from philosophy and religion to botany and medicine, focus upon the nervous system provided a further and decisive step in the undaunted march of the reductionist-mechanist approach, by separating his views on the nature of the mind from what he was able to deduce from practical experience. He thus reduced the whole into properties or parts in an attempt to explain the complex nature of the nervous system. [61, 62] Coupled with the work of Luigi Galvani (1737-1798), who confirmed the relationship between nerve impulses and electric current, the eighteenth century also witnessed the birth of another reductionist science, neurophysiology. [63] Other workers of the time such as the Reverend Stephen Hales inserted glass tubes into the arteries and veins of horses to produce one of the first studies of blood pressure, in an attempt to explain the actual workings of the animal body.

Specialization and the compartmentalization of medical knowledge

Medicine in the age of Enlightenment also witnessed the rise of other specializations or what might be called "the systemization of the reductionist-mechanist model in epistemology." Anonia Giuseppe Testa (1756-1814) formalized the discipline of cardiology; the work of Nils Von Rosenstein (1706-1773) and George Armstrong (1720-1789) fostered pediatrics as a separate domain of study; Paul Gottfired Werlhof (1699-1767) inspired the discipline of hematology; the work of Philippe Pinel (1745-1826), Jean Esquirol (1772-1840), and Wilhelm Greisinger (1817-1868) provided a taxonomy and anatomicopathological classification of mental diseases and stimulated the formal discipline of psychiatry. [64] Surgery was given a whole new impetus in France where the first Royal Academy of Surgery was chartered in 1731, thereby distinguishing the tradition of medical surgeons from the barber-surgeons. Conjoined with developments in anatomy and physiology, surgery became a manual art of reductionist distinction. Surgery also prospered in England with famous surgeons such as William Cheselden (1688-1752), Percivall Pott (1714-1788), and the famed Scotsman John Hunter, who is acclaimed as having an experimental foundation for surgery based upon a set of coherent principles drawn from the biological sciences. [65] Perhaps the greatest contribution of the eighteenth century to the reductionist-mechanist medical orientation was the discovery of vaccination. It was of course the English physician Edward Jenner (1749-1823) who noticed that milkmaids contracted cowpox but never smallpox. On the suspicion that the milkmaids had developed an immunity to smallpox, he decided to inoculate a small boy with the inoculate vaccine obtained from a milkmaid afflicted with cowpox. When the boy was later inoculated with smallpox, he failed to contract the disease, though he did develop a mild exanthema. With the resounding success of vaccination, the reductionist thesis seemed to be incontrovertible. Disease was reduced to one causative agent with one specific treatment. [66, 67] It was a reasonable assumption that the body was invaded by something which caused a disease such as smallpox. However, despite Leeuwenhoek's description of bacteria in 1683 it was not until Otto Muller (1730-1784) made a systematic description of different types of bacteria that the link between specific microorganisms and specific disease was made. [68] The battle against disease came thus to be fought at the microscopic level, microbe against microbe. The concept of disease as a malfunction of the parts within the human machine took on a far more sophisticated interpretation, but the interpretation was still mechanistic. While it was conceded that the human body was more complicated than Descartes' mechanical image of the works of a clock, the basic commitment to a reductionist explanation of biological functions through the analysis of the whole into the electrical and chemical interactions of its fundamental parts preserved the spirit of the Cartesian paradigm in subtler mechanistic terms.

By the nineteenth century the vast literature which had accumulated from areas such as anatomy and physiology served to afford researchers an unprecedented knowledge of the human body even in its finest details. Spurred in part by this knowledge and the steady improvements made to the microscope, originally a seventeenth-century invention, the advent of microbiology represented the next major development in the evolution of reductionist methodology, because it allowed the whole to be reduced not only to organs and tissues but to individual cells and ultimately to organelles within each cell. The study of microbiology gave rise to two prominent research directions: cell biology and bacteriology. It was Robert Hooke who is reputed to have coined the term "cell" to describe the minute structures which appeared when viewing the body microscopically. Although a number of researchers were engaged in studies which involved the analysis of cells, no integrated theory of biological functions in cellular terms was formulated until the nineteenth century.

Taking Morgagni's notion of gross lesions in organs leading to disease, Xavier Bichat (1771-1802) examined and divided the organs of the body into twenty-one "membranes" or "tissues." He compared the structure of the body to a woven fabric or web and, from the Greek *histos* (web), the new method of *histology* for studying the structure of the body emerged. [69]

It was the genius of Rudolf Virchow (1821-1902) that established "histology" in the sense of a formal science of cell biology. According to Virchow, the cell was the fundamental structural component in the human body and the explanation of disease could not be understood apart from it. Regarding disease pathology as abnormal cell physiology, he postulated structural alterations, deformities, and other cellular irregularities as the explanation of disease. [70, 71] Where Morgagni had used the distinction between normal and pathological anatomy as the lineage of disease to a structural pathology of *organal* ancestry, and Bichat to tissues, Virchow used the distinction to continue the reduction to an even lower level of analysis, the cell. Virchow's work provided the foundations for a new concept of disease and for the science of histopathology which would promulgate it. Virchow's research inspired the publication of the first book on histology, written by the Swiss Rudolf Albert von Kolliker (1817-1905), in which disease was construed on the analogy of a civil war between germs and leucocytes, the leucocytes representing the police force of the cell state.[72] Strongly influenced by Virchow and dubbed the Vesalius of histology, the romantic German revolutionary agitator Jacob Henle (1809-1895) laid the foundations of modern epidemiology on similar reductionist ground.[73]

The evolution of the reductionist paradigm found its other expression in perhaps the most celebrated nineteenth-century contribution to medical progress, the aetiopathic or "germ theory of disease." Anticipated in *obiter dicta* by scientists such as Father Athanasius Kircher (1602-1680), Enrico Acerbi (1785-1827), and Agostina Bassi (1773-1856), the endeavor to link microbes of bacteria with disease culminated in the research of Pasteur, Koch, and von Behring. [74, 75, 76] Concerned to save the French wine and dairy industries from ruin, Louis Pasteur (1822-1895) discovered that lactic and butyric fermentation of alcohols were caused by either aerobic (oxygen requiring) or anaerobic (non-oxygen requiring) bacteria. Having identified bacteria as the cause of fermentation of wine, he determined that if they could be destroyed by some process such as sufficiently raising the temperature of the wine (pasteurization) the wine could be preserved. Proving that bacteria were not the consequence of fermentation but its cause, and that they came from the air, water, and earth, he had solved the ancient conundrum of *contagium animatum* by postulating the bacteriological origins of contagious disease. Pasteur is of course remembered also for having saved the French silk industry by discovering the cause of pebrine, the silkworm disease. He is also famed for his use of the inoculation with attenuated viruses and vaccines to protect chickens and swine from anthrax (splenic fever) and cholera. Pasteur continued his work with attenuated viruses and overcame the dreaded rabies in 1885. He is known to have investigated the use of penicillin some seventy years before the work of Sir Alexander Fleming on the same subject.

It was Robert Koch (1843-1910) however who postulated and formalized the reductionist nexus between specific diseases and the species of germs which caused them. His identification of the particular bacteriological origins of tuberculosis represented yet another triumph for the methodology of reductionism and provided a practical example of the concept of microbic specificity. Koch eventually went on to articulate a set of criteria by reference to which it could be demonstrated whether any particular correlation between specific diseases and their specific causes was correct. [77, 78, 79, 80] Koch's "postulates," as the set of criteria has come to be known, have been included in the curriculum syllabus of medical schools ever since. In addition to the foregoing medical achievements Koch endeavored to enunciate a methodology of disinfection, to trace the germ etiology of tuberculosis, and to plot the developmental patterns of wound infections.

One of Koch's pupils, Emil von Behring (1854-1917), continued the work of his much-emulated teacher and succeeded in discovering that while invasive bacteria in the body secrete toxins, the body produces antitoxins as a measure in its defense against them. Consistent with this research orientation, his greatest success came in the development of an antitoxin for diphtheria, an achievement for which he earned the Nobel Prize in Medicine in 1901, four years prior to the award of the same prize to his beloved teacher in 1905.

Another significant contributor to the discipline of bacteriology was Edwin Klebs (1834-1913) whose immense distinction derived in part from his discovery of the diphtheria virus, finally isolated by Freidrich Joffler (1852-1915). He is perhaps best known, however, for having plotted the medical geography, so to say, of the "empire" of syphilis by inoculating anthropoid apes with the germ. Another reductionist success came with the invention of the technique of chromotherapy which in fact set the stage for chemotherapy. Fascinated by the discrimination patterns and general selectivity of dyes for particular types of tissue, Paul Ehrlich (1854-1915) set himself the task of isolating dyes with an intense chemical affinity for particular bacteria. His quest for "therapy by colors" was eventually transformed into the search for "magic bullets" or substances capable of destroying specific microbes without degrading the cell in which they were located. His production of an arsenical drug (Salvarsan) was the first chemical compound used successfully to treat a specific infection (in this case, syphilis). A few years later he developed the drug, Neosalvarsan, a less toxic arsenic-based drug also used in the fight against syphilis.[81, 82]

In 1922 Harold Raistrick initiated the study of the metabolic secretions of molds which were antimicrobial in their effect, but the age of antibiotics is not reckoned to have begun until 1939-1940, when Rene Dubos discovered thyrotricin and demonstrated that microbial metabolism could be deliberately inhibited and impeded.[83] Although Alexander Fleming first discovered penicillin in 1928 when he noticed the degradation of *Staphylococcus* cultures brought about airborne molds, it was not until 1941 that the publication of the clinical results of numerous tests on penicillin, establishing its low toxicity and antimicrobial effect, brought the drug to the attention of the medical profession.[84]

By the close of the nineteenth century the "germ theory of disease" virtually dominated the methodology of medical science. Despite the significant contribution of the physiologist Claude Bernard (1813-1878) and the school of cell biology built upon his views, the highly reductionist concept of disease-specific etiology became progressively entrenched. Bernard had stressed the functional correlation of the internal organs and the unity of the various physicochemical processes within the human organism, suggesting that disease could best be explicated by reference to disruptions in their equilibrium. Rather than tracing disease to a specific germ cause as Koch had done, Bernard was convinced that disease resulted from a constellation of factors, including environmental ones, acting concurrently to upset the internal balance of the living system. [85] The germ theory of disease gained adherents in a way that Bernard's less reductionist approach did not for a number of reasons. In addition to having an articulate spokesman, Pasteur, to argue on behalf of the etiological theory, using epidemics current in Europe at the time as examples of the germ theory, the doctrine of specific disease causation was consonant with the underlying philosophy of reductio-mechanism underpinning nineteenth-century science. It has been suggested, for example, that the Linnean classification of living forms, accepted at the beginning of the century, provided a ready model to be extrapolated to the analysis and classification of disease. Having already adopted the concept of a taxonomy of plants and animals, the idea of a taxonomy of diseases was simply a natural extension of the accepted reductionist classification of nature in general. [86]

Other nineteenth-century developments in medicine both reinforced and reflected the reductionist-mechanist philosophy of nature. The invention of the stethoscope, the endoscope, the bronchoscope, X-rays, and devices for taking blood pressure, along with the newly developed techniques biopsy, esophagoscopy and pyelography permitted the visualization and examination of internal parts of the living body hitherto inaccessible to the medical eye. The substratum of medicine became more physicochemical and physiological, giving a new importance to the role of mensuration in diagnosis and treatment. The introduction of charts, the pocket clinical thermometer, case histories of the course of the disease, and tables portraying changes and comparisons of functional signs gave reductionist medicine a ritualistic formality that enhanced its impact. Neurology was advanced by Duchene's electrological treatment of nervous diseases, and by Turck of Vienna who located the center of articulated speech. [87]

Psychiatry required its autonomy and was established as an independent science. Reductionist philosophy of medicine inspired an organic approach to mental illness, especially with the investigative work of Antoine Bayle (1799-1858) into the cause of general paralysis of the insane. Bayle held this condition to be due to chronic meningitis. [88] The final proof of the cause came in 1913 when Hideyo Noguchi (1876-1928) announced paralysis of the insane to be caused by the spirochete which causes syphilis. [89] Contrasted with this organic approach to mental illness is the psychological approach of Phillipe Pinel (1745-1826), famed for the introduction of humane treatment for the insane, and his followers, including Jean Esquirol (1772-1840) who introduced the concept of depression and other non-organic factors as contributing to mental illness. [90] For the most part, however, correlations and classifications were made between neuropsychiatric symptoms and their causes in brain lesions, in the cell architecture of the brain and congenital deformations, and in vocological entities. Emil Kraeplin (1856-1926) attempted quite successfully to sort out the confusion between the theories by distinguishing between "endogenic" and "symptomatic" mental diseases. [91] The concept of mental infirmity as a manifestation of a somatic disease was made explicit by Alois Alzheimer (1864-1915) and Franz Nissl (1860-1919), and the basic notion that all mental disorders have organic causes admitting of organic treatment defined the reductionist methodology of psychiatry. [92] Indeed, it was partly in reaction to this uncompromisingly dogmatic reduction that the psychological approach to mental disease was initiated. The work, for example, of Sigmund Freud (1856-1939), a Viennese physician, was directed towards a more comprehensive science of mind than the organic etiology of mental illness allowed. Freud's somewhat revolutionary methods had shown that unpleasant repressed experiences could disturb the equilibrium of health, and led to the widespread practice of psychoanalysis.

Research into aphasia (absence of or difficulty with speech) exemplifies the reduction of medicine and psychiatry. Determined to reduce aphasia to a mental disorder, Pierre Broca (1824-1880) localized the speech center to the left temporal lobe of the brain, and believed that lesions there gave rise to aphasia. [93] Hughlings Jackson (1835-1911) and his followers H.C. Bastian (1837-1915) and Henry Head (1861-1940) on the other hand believed that other regions of the brain such as auditory and visual word centers were also involved. [94] Head in 1926 concluded that a speech defect was involved with higher intellect and related to disturbances in symbolic formulation. Both groups, however, still affirm a reductionist approach by splitting the whole brain into ever-reduced parts in an attempt to understand the whole.

By the turn of the twentieth century the reductionist-mechanist paradigm literally dominated the conceptual framework within the evolution and continued development of medical science took place. While the Cartesian model extended the concept of the 'body-machine' far beyond anything imagined by the Greeks, the advent of twentieth-century nuclear physics served to extend the concept of reductionism to depths of reality unimagined by Descartes. In little more than a century the reductionist account of the etiology had shifted from its seat in diseased organs to the tissues of such organs and on to the cells of the tissues, from the cells of the body to the microscopic bacteria or germs which infest and disrupt them. Finally, in the twentieth century the reduction would be taken one step further.

Nuclear medicine, drugs and 'gene-dreaming healing'

Revolutionized on the one hand by Max Planck's formulation of quantum action and on the other by Albert Einstein's theory of general relativity, the natural sciences took mechanism to the depths of the atom and beyond. Quantum theory entailed the radical reconceptualization of matter, while relativity theory entailed the radical unification of space, time, and gravitation. There is at present no comprehensive and consistent formulation of a theory of unification for these two developments, though much current research within physics is directed towards this aim. Inasmuch as certain of these issues will be directly addressed later in the book, it would be extraneous to our present consideration to pursue them here. Suffice to say that on both accounts, the principles of reduction are extreme and provide a new reductionist base for the technologization of medicine.

The understanding of biological phenomena, on the nuclear model of reductionism, proceeds to the molecular and atomic level of analysis. The bacteriological and microchemical orientation, for example, is given a new foundation in the technological capacity provided by the electron microscope (invented by Busch in 1926) to examine atomic structures as they pertain to disease. Utilizing the technology of nuclear medicine, biochemical lesions, viruses, collagen diseases, and a host of other illnesses are studied by way of the analysis of their atomic components. Reinforcing the nuclear reductionist trend and often resulting from it have been innovations in diagnostic methods such as electrophoresis, microspectrophotometry, stratigraphic radiography, tomography, ventriculography, and electromyography. The electrocardiograph was introduced by Einthoven in 1903, the electroencephalograph in 1929 by Berger, Shindler's gastroscope in 1932, ballistocardiography in 1939 by Starr, and the cyclone knife by O'Brien and McKinley in 1943. [95] The specialty of atomic medicine which employs radioactivity to destroy diseased tissues and inhibit the proliferation of cellular malignancies has produced a range of devices peculiar to its own enterprise. Cancerous tumors, for example, have been treated by a device called an "atomic pistol" which "shoots" or injects radioactive gold "bullets" into them. Radioisotopes in solution can also be similarly injected. Another innovation was the radioactive lamp designed to direct radioactive cobalt rays on tissue specifically designated as cancerous. The influence of twentieth-century physics has also been felt in biochemistry where the emphasis upon atomic processes such as chain reactions, catalytic actions, and isotopy exemplifies the methodological commitment of medical science to nuclear reductionism.

Technological advances in medicine have also contributed to the reductionist orientation in twentieth-century surgery. Surgical techniques were themselves enormously improved, partly as a consequence of the growth of medical knowledge drawing from anatomy and physiology, and partly from the depth and range of experience gained from two world wars. Improvements in anesthesiology have afforded surgeons more time to reduce the physiological trauma to patients and to perfect their surgical procedures. The discovery of antibiotics, which derived largely from Pasteur's earlier research in bacteriology, was also a major factor in increasing the success rate of surgical operations. Armed with antibiotics which prevented infection, anticoagulants and antihemorrhagic drugs which controlled bleeding and blood changes, vitamins (named in 1906 by Casimis Funk) to prevent malnutrition, and mineral salts to prevent dehydration, surgeons were able to usher in a whole new era in surgery. [96] They were also assisted by other types of technological developments, tools, and devices. Scalpels were especially designed and adapted to meet the particular requirements of different surgical procedures. Other diagnostic techniques such as radioactive tracers, ultrasound, and radar detectors for isolating specific organic processes proved to be invaluable. Microsurgical techniques were developed, bone-replacements with materials foreign to the body made possible, and innovations using the laser beam invented. The classification of blood into three main groups served to ensure the possibility of successful blood transfusions. Artificial organs have been transplanted, and in 1960 the first transplantation of a human heart was carried out by Christian Barnard, followed by a spate of organ transplants of varying degrees of success. All of these techniques reinforce the reductio-mechanistic paradigm—the human body is a machine which can be reduced to its parts which in turn, with the twentieth-century allopathic medicine, can be replaced.

The progression of biology to the nuclear level has been accompanied also by the discovery of intracellular viruses, microsomes, and the molecular structure and function of the gene. The focus of molecular biology upon the gene, in particular, is of enormous importance philosophically, for it signifies the culmination of the reductionist quest in the twentieth century for the basic building-blocks of all life. The implications of this view for the philosophy of medicine are equally momentous, for reductionist genetics gives rise to the false impression that all biological functions can be understood in terms of molecular mechanisms at the genetic level. Genetic engineering in turn represents the scientific way in which these mechanisms and the diseases for which they are responsible can be manipulated and controlled. Inasmuch as genetic engineering also betrays the convert commitment of science to reductionist epistemology, a commitment to be elucidated in a later chapter, some discussion of its evolution and development may be apposite here.

For the origin of the principles underpinning genetic engineering, the reference is to an Austrian monk of the nineteenth century, Gregor Mendel, whose study of the inheritance patterns of the ordinary garden pea is regarded as having established the science of genetics. It was the Swiss scientist Johann Miescher, however, who while investigating the nucleus of living cells discovered an acidic compound with some of the peculiar properties attributed to DNA (deoxyribonucleic acid). Despite the flirtation of the concept of DNA as a genetic construct, its role in transmitting inherited characteristics would defy analysis until well into the twentieth century.

During the first half of the twentieth century it was determined that all living cells were composed of protein and nucleic acids, combined in complicated chainlike structures whose exact form and mechanics were yet to be revealed. Once it was realized that cells also contain another constituent, i.e., the agents called "enzymes" capable of promoting particular types of chemical reactions within the cell, it was soon demonstrated that every such reaction is determined by the presence of a particular enzyme. Working in the 1930s with cellular extracts of killed bacteria, Oswald Avery and his co-workers were convinced that there was a *transforming factor* in all cells capable of passing on genetic information from one cell or organism to another: this factor they postulated was DNA. In 1941 came the discovery by Beadle and Tatum that the synthesis of enzymes was a process controlled by the genes and thus that hereditary traits are themselves dependent upon the genetic program specifying the synthesis of those enzymes which instantiate one genetic trait rather than another. [97] Despite these rich insights, the structure of the gene, a nucleo-protein, and the structure of the enzyme, itself a protein constellation, remained a mystery. Within two decades, however, the genetic code was broken and the molecular structure of genes and enzymes made transparent. With this new knowledge came an understanding of the chemical mechanisms involved in gene replication, mutation, and the synthesis of protein. In 1950 Linus Pauling elucidated the secondary structure of the protein molecule, introducing the model of a coiled pattern in the shape of either a left-handed or right-handed alpha helix as a heuristic description of a sector of the amino acid sequence of which it is composed. [98, 99] The idea of a coiled helix had considerable explanatory power, and it was adapted by the researchers James Watson and Francis Crick to reveal the structure of DNA itself, the genetic material in the chromosomes. The results of their investigations came to public light in 1953 with the publication of their celebrated article on this topic in the scientific journal *Nature,* and their breakthrough was soon hailed as marking the inception of the genetic revolution. [100, 101]

In that article Watson and Crick reported that the microscopic structure of DNA had the form of a helix not unlike Pauling's protein molecule, but in this case it was the model of a twisting double helix resembling a spiral staircase. The steps of the spiral staircase were constituted by what were called "base units." Differences in genetic makeup, they claimed, depended upon the particular arrangement of base units which comprised a modest sequence of four chemical nucleotide (i.e., adenine, guanine, cytosine, and thymine). Often abbreviated by their first letters AGCT, these chemical substances have come to be called the "genetic alphabet." Arranging the four letters in as many different configurations as possible, it was observed that there were sixty-four possible combinations, more than a sufficient number to produce the twenty fundamental amino acids which in turn combine in a multitude of sequences to produce the entire spectrum of protein variations manifest in living things. [102] Generally speaking, the smaller the number of genes in combination, the simpler the form of the individual organisms and vice versa.

Within a decade of their original discovery Watson and Crick had also unraveled the mystery surrounding the basic mechanism through which DNA carries out self-replication and protein synthesis, thereby uncovering the process by which genetic information is encoded in the chromosomes. Their discovery was highly illuminating and paved the way for future developments in genetic engineering by showing *how* the genetic properties and traits of all living organisms, regardless how complex, were encoded by the same chemical substances and governed by an identifiable code script. Nirenberg and Matthaei of the National Institutes of Health, in testing the messenger RNA hypothesis, proved the specific base coding for several amino acids and made available a method for defining other amino acids. [103] Having broken the genetic code, it was at least in principle possible to undertake systematically the reconstruction or engineering of specific hereditary characteristics within a particular genotype.

While the study of genes and their structure reinforces the reductionist notion of being able to understand the whole only in terms of its reduced parts, the work of Jacob and Monod is antireductionist, and confirms the idea of the whole being indeed greater than the sum of its parts. Working at the Pasteur Institute in Paris, Jacob and Monod introduced the concept of regulation of genes. Their work showed that genes will only synthesize enzymes when required by the cell, thus introducing the notion of structural and regulator genes. [104]

It was not until the 1970s, however, that the most radical and revolutionary development in genetic engineering occurred. To understand why it was truly revolutionary, the technology it deploys needs to be contrasted with the traditional concept of gene manipulation. In a manner of speaking the concept of genetic engineering, indeed its practice is not really new. Since the beginning of history, there have been persistent attempts to change and improve the quality of nature's cornucopia of living organisms. Farmers have long been engaged, for example, in the selective breeding of animals, the discriminate planting of some grains and not others, and the hybridization of fruits and vegetables. There have throughout ages been attempts or proposals to manipulate the human gene pool through the selective breeding of humans. Hitler's' program of positive eugenics is a case in point, though the notion of prohibiting or at least of discouraging marriage and the reproduction of children for individuals of incompatible blood types, or who might be carriers of certain inheritable diseases, in not as uncommon as one might think.

Although we have throughout the ages sought to engineer particular genetic variations within species, there was until the 1970's no technology available to permit the engineering of the genotype of the species themselves. Moreover, the genetic boundaries between any two genotypes have been virtually insoluble and inexorably distinct, before this time. All this has now changed. For the first time in the history of the human race we have procured, through reductionist technology, power over our own evolution. It is now possible to engineer the genetic inheritance of an individual by recombining DNA from altogether different organisms, thereby introducing new gene traits to replace the old. In the early 1970s Herbert Boyer of the University of California and Stanly Cohen of Stanford University succeeded in stitching together slices of genetic material from two completely unrelated species, thus creating a new biological form of life. [105] Referred to as "recombinant DNA technology," this radically innovative form of genetic engineering revolutionized medical practice, and reshaped our concepts of health and healing. For instance, it is now possible to transfer genetic characteristics from one genus of living organism to another and even to edit the genetic code of an individual by reprogramming gene patterns which would otherwise have been absolute and unalterable. Although not a feature of this piece, we have in recent times been witness to the editing of the genetic characteristics of plants. Tomatoes, for example, have been marked with the genetic material of a fish, hence providing new qualities such as the ability to resist frost. [106] This example, despite its relevance to other forms of life, may at some point in the future represent the dynamic influence genetic engineering can have on the living organism of the human species.

Genetic engineering and the ultra-reductionist philosophical principles that undergird it slipped almost imperceptibly into the theory and practice of twentieth-century medicine. Committed to a methodology which seeks to eradicate disease by manipulating the biological mechanisms through which disease operates, medical researchers have found in genetic engineering the promise of exposing the ultimate context of manipulation in respect of every mechanism within the body, including the mechanisms which determine immune responses. [107] For example, as is the case with a type of human genetic engineering known as somatic therapy, we are already witness to children born with severe combined immune deficiency (SCID) now living a healthy life that would otherwise have not been the case without such technology available. [108]

In addition to the proposed benefits which genetic engineering affords for the screening and control of genetic disorders responsible for mental disease, it can also be combined with IVF techniques in the service of gene therapy. By making the genetic material of the zygote accessible for manipulation, IVF facilitates the process of both genetic screening and gene transfer at an early enough stage in embryonic development that the introduction of non-defective DNA can be incorporated into the germ-line (sex) cells as part of the normal integrative and developmental process. Although gene therapy is in principle possible at later stages of development, including adulthood, the ability to direct nondefective genes for integration into the specific community of chromosomes which manifest the defect becomes progressively more difficult as cell structure becomes progressively more differentiated, witnessed in recent times by scientist testing gene transfer on children with muscular dystrophy. [109] The alternative procedure, however, of removing from the body a sample of the defective cell population for recombinant therapy, to be subsequently returned to the body for assimilation, is an area in the field still being perfected. [110]

Given the ostensible aim of health for all, promoted by a growing body of health authorities worldwide, the use of genetic engineering as a medical tool for eradicating the disabling, disfiguring, and deadly diseases of our society would seem *prima facie* to be entirely warranted. Who would not wish to see the end of the diminution of the crippling diseases of mind and body which are genetically caused? Advocates of human genetic engineering extol its virtue, and the public is encouraged to believe that its use in medicine is not only right but that any attempt to inhibit this development would be irresponsible and wrong.

There is in all this, however, a deeper philosophical issue which the glamour and rhetoric of genetic engineering can inadvertently hide. Genetic engineering is not just another technological foray capable of making a contribution to medical science. Genetic engineering signals the culmination of the reductionist-mechanist disposition in medical science. It is the technology which defines implicitly the way in which we conceptualize our relationship with nature. Genetic engineering represents the final transition in the desacrilization of nature and of ourselves, for the unit of integrity is no longer defined by the identity of the species or its members by the anonymity of the gene. What is lost in the reduction from the organism itself to the genes which define it is the identity of the whole being, which is something more than the aggregate representative of its genetic components. Since there is nothing sacred about a gene, so the argument goes, there is nothing blasphemous about manipulating it. Species boundaries are illusory, for the fundamental unit of life is not the species or its individual members but the genes which in different ways but equally define them all. [111] It is this philosophy which legitimizes the proposals to transfer from one species to another the chemical signatures encoded in the genes of each. In the reductionist scenario the common denominator of all life is DNA and thus the gene pool of all living organisms which it enshrines. Just as we have desacralized and exploited the non-living resources of the earth by reducing the things of the earth to the things of which they are made, so we exploit the living things of the earth by reducing them to a gene pool which itself becomes a resource to be exploited. The philosophical relevance for medicine of genetic engineering as the scientific development which rivals the discovery of nuclear energy in the present cultural epoch is that the reductionist-mechanist rationale which inspired both is in the end inimical to health.

It is to be admitted that from the beginning of history, we have engineered the structure of nature and tailored the fiber of its raw materials to suit our needs. Less inclined to recant our indiscretions, however, what we have often failed to admit is that we have not always engineered it for the better. Our lust for power over nature, combined with our reverence for the reductionist-mechanist technology of science which has served to express it, have led to a pathetic degradation of the world around us. We have treated the world as if it were a machine whose parts can be used up and replaced at will. Our hapless engineering of nature has finally brought about a man-made holocaust of unprecedented dimensions. Our cities and surrounding areas are drenched in acid rain, our lakes and streams polluted, our drinking water increasingly less fit for consumption, our farmlands converted into chemical waste dumps, and the earth itself denuded by the loss of nearly one-third of its prime topsoil, due largely to the ravaging of its forests and plants. Now that we have distorted and disfigured the environment so as to make it almost unlivable and certainly unhealthy we turn to genetic engineering to help us distort ourselves so that we can adjust to the world we have distorted. Moreover, our genetic adjustments are sponsored on the pretense that it is not we but our biological imperfections which will be eliminated. In the next chapter it will be argued that despite the technological achievements of medical science, there is a crisis in medicine which is in large part due to the reductionist-mechanist philosophy which underpins those achievements.

Summary

Before proceeding to the next chapter let us draw together into a coherent whole the sundry historical facets of the conceptual evolution of the reduction-mechanist model in medicine. The process of disease and the craft of healing, we observed, have been a part of the history of the human race for longer than its history has been recorded. Although there is no simple logical progression in the development of the philosophical underpinnings of modern medicine, a general progression towards reductionism can nevertheless be discerned.

The nexus between medicine and religion, and medicine and philosophy, has been historically manifest in the social roles played by witch doctors, shamans, wisemen, priests and priestesses, and even the beings designated by the ancients as the gods and goddesses of healing. Within this nexus the craft of healing was almost always more than the mechanical manipulation of the body, whether by means of bone-setting, primitive surgery, or herbalism. Disease was commonly regarded as the result of sin or apostasy and the mode of its eradication as repentance and self-flagellation. Despite their naiveté, primitive healers often seemed unconsciously aware, however, of the need to represent their contributions to healing in terms of the mental and physical dimensions of the human organism. The ancient craft of healing was not so much a separate activity as an activity incorporated into and expressed by the entire religious or philosophical belief system of the time. The craft of healing was thus socially mediated through the conventions, taboos, rituals, patterns of organization, and catechisms of spiritual guidance.

By the time of the early Egyptians and Babylonians the initial break between religion and medicine as signaled by the partitioning of shamanic duties into herbalist treatments of illness on the one hand and magico-religious treatments of illness attended by priests and priestesses on the other. With the advent of the Hippocratic School, medicine had virtually succeeded in throwing off its religious heritage, and the concept of disease as sin was replaced by Hippocrates's theory of the four humors, which explained disease as a natural process and traced it causally to disruptions of the internal balance of these elements. Hippocrates's recognition of the importance of preventive medicine, hygiene, diet, the environment, and the life of virtue in the promotion of health marked one of the most innovative and revolutionary developments in the history of medicine. Health and virtue were reckoned as two sides of the same coin, for health and disease were on the Hippocratic view a function of lifestyle. Because the Hippocratic physician was primarily an itinerant healer, however, the practical application of Hippocrates's views by those who followed him focused upon quick and accurate diagnosis, combined with interventionist techniques using herbs, drugs, and even surgery. In practical terms the idea of preserving the delicate equilibrium associated with the internal harmony of the humors gave way to the causal theory of disease implicit in it. The notion that disease could be explained in terms of material causes within the body was endorsed and elaborated by the Romans, whose interventionist techniques included an increasing reliance upon surgery. Galen's anatomic concept of disease encouraged the study of anatomy though vivisection, which in turn reinforced the development of the surgical tradition.

With the fall of the Roman Empire and the destruction of the Library at Alexandria the inchoate tradition of western medical science was thrown into chaos. Partly as a result of the Moorish school of medicine, the late Middle Ages witnessed a revival of the causal theory of medicine, coupled with a mechanist view of the body, and gave birth to hospitals for the practice of medicine, and universities for the training of at least some of those who would practice it. Universities also provided an important environment and catalyst for medical research and the formulation of medical theory. The theoretic momentum of this period was carried forward and expanded in the Renaissance with a renewed interest in anatomy, coupled with a new interest in the individual diseases of the age (e.g., exanthematic typhus, diphtherial angina, and syphilis) and the specific nature of their causes. The concept of diseases as actual entities which invade the body was introduced by Paracelsus during this period. Surgical procedures also became more successful as the detailed anatomical sketches by men such as Leonardo de Vinci were used to advance medical understanding of the intricate workings of the human body. The persistent commitment to the causal theory of disease led medical researchers to search for the fundamental elements within the body upon which it relied.

It was in the seventeenth century that Descartes' mechanistic philosophy was coupled with the methodology of reductionism to revolutionize the approach to medical theory and practice. His work benefitted, as we saw, from the work of Galileo, and was later embellished by Newton, whose reductionist method of quantification has been a cornerstone of medical science ever since. With the development of the microscope, things too small to be observed by the naked eye, and previously only conjectured to exist, were subsumed as quantifiable variables within the reductionist methodology, and the latrophysicists boldly proclaimed that the body was merely a machine. As a result of Harvey's demonstration of the circulation of blood, and Riolan and Pecquet's confirmation of lymphatic circulation, both physiology and anatomy were put on a new reductio-mechanistic footing.

With the proliferation of medical journals in the eighteenth century, the rate of new medical discoveries increased exponentially. Digitalis was introduced by Withering in the treatment of dropsy, angina pectoris was depicted by Heberden, the physiology of respiration revealed by Lavorisier, and the discovery of smallpox made by Jenner, thus initiating the trend towards vaccination. Medical science in the nineteenth century, it will be recalled from our survey, relied upon a research methodology progressively dominated by the canons of reductio-mechanistic philosophy and the corresponding technology to which it gave rise. Improvements made to the microscope complimented and inspired the cell theory of disease and also led to the even more successful germ theory of disease, for which Pasteur, Koch, and Behring have become so well-known. Surgery was literally propelled forward with the discovery of surgical anesthesia, and specialization led to advances in obstetrics, ophthalmology, and gynecology, to name a few. The substratum of medicine became more physiological and more physicochemical in orientation, and neuropathology gained a foothold as finer and finer aspects of bodily mechanisms were required to satisfy the reductionist quest for etiological ultimacy.

The vast array of technological developments in twentieth-century medicine, we observed, have been spectacular. The dominance of the reductio-mechanist paradigm has perhaps been most conspicuous in the area of nuclear medicine on the one hand and molecular biology (with special reference to genetic engineering) on the other. On the nuclear medical model, disease is reduced to its manifestations at the level of atomic structures, as are the new forms of medical treatment which it engenders. Technological developments in the twentieth century, such as the invention of the electron microscope, reinforced reductionism by providing a route of observational access into the subatomic domain for which there was previously no entry. With the new and deeper level of analysis came not only new specializations such as nuclear medicine, but also new approaches to anatomy, physiology, and biology.

The shift of emphasis from biology in general to molecular biology in particular has led in the second half of this century to the discovery of the technological innovations associated with genetic engineering, the culmination philosophically of the reductionist disposition in biology. One of the central assumptions underpinning genetic engineering is that the proliferation of all life forms, including bacteria and viruses, can be explained by reference to a universal code-script whose variant internal combinations define the nature of the resultant biological organisms. DNA represents the fundamental building-blocks, not just of *human* life, but of *all* life. With regard to medical science the assumption is that all disease processes are fundamentally organic processes, and that inasmuch as DNA determines the nature of *all* organic processes, the ability to manipulate and control DNA is tantamount to being able to manipulate and control disease. The common denominator of all disease, on this view, is DNA, and thus the gene pool in its entirety stands philosophically as the ultimate medical resource. Genetic engineering, however, signals more than just the culmination of biological reductionism in science; it is a powerful symbol and reflection of the reductio-mechanist theory of knowledge which set the context for its discovery.

We labor this point because it is a central contention of this book that the reductio-mechanistic disposition in medical science is part and parcel of a theory of knowledge which defines our relationship to nature in terms which we contend are inimical to the advancement of health. This is one major reason why we do not believe that the resolution of the crisis in health care is to be found in more 'high-technology' medicine, for it is in part the philosophical commitment to high technology which is precisely the origin of the crisis. If there is to be a new vision of health care, it is essential that the framework of its interpretation is not itself epistemically myopic. We are convinced that the continued commitment of allopathic medicine to the reductio-mechanistic methodology of scientism and its accompanying epistemology will only serve to perpetuate and indeed exacerbate the very health problems for which we as a society are seeking resolutions. The time has now come to elaborate this charge, and it is to this task that we must now turn in the subsequent chapter.

CHAPTER 2

Scientism and the catastrophe of the modern health system

The ascendancy of scientism in contemporary society is a phenomenon whose full impact upon our thought and culture, including the nature of medical theory and practice, has become increasingly difficult to assess. The genesis of the complexity is itself difficult to assess, since the criteria of assessment are themselves scientific. The assessment afforded thus suffers the malady of being conceptually infected by the very reductionist assumptions with which assessment we seek. An account of the contribution which scientism makes to our understanding of the world, for example, will almost unavoidably be judged by an understanding of the world which is itself scientific. Either the circularity is not noticed, or it is acknowledged on the ground that it does not really matter, inasmuch as scientism provides a genuinely scientific understanding of the world, to be preferred to any other such understanding. On interpretation the assumption stands that the more scientific medicine becomes, the 'better' or more effective it is. Implicit in the historical evolution of the bioreductionist model to which we have referred in the previous chapter is just an assumption. Committed to medical progress, researchers have been duped into believing that the problems confronting conventional medicine can be overcome by relying upon the very conceptual scheme of reductionist science and its accompanying technology whose continued implementation serves unwittingly to proliferate them.

The general burden of this chapter is to show that as a consequence of its progressive reliance upon medical scientism, western medicine is in a state of crisis and of transition. The nature of the crisis is becoming increasingly clear, but the direction of the transition remains confused. One predominant reason for the confusion lies in having recognized the signs of crisis without having exposed the roots of the restrictive philosophical system out of which it has arisen. One direction of the transition thus leads to what we will call the "technological fallacy" or the belief that improved and more sophisticated medical technology will make everything better, including the things which, by dint of its sophistication, improved medical technology is by its very nature bound to make worse. The main burden of the present chapter will be to illustrate three aspects of the fallacy.

1. High-technology, bioreductionist medicine does not provide a form of health care which is cost-effective.
2. Medical science can no more be justifiably blamed for the growing incidence of chronic and degenerative diseases such as cardiovascular disease and cancer than it can be justifiably praised for the virtual eradication of infectious diseases such as typhoid fever and smallpox. The truth is that the effects of medical intervention on The advancement of community health have been negligible and in large part irrelevant.
3. Far from succeeding in advancing community health, the interventionist orientation of bioreductionist medicine has paradoxically contributed to its demise by creating additional illness as a result of its intervention. Consideration will thus be given to the category of ill health known as " iatrogenic" (i.e., physician-and hospital-caused) illness; and the category will be expanded to show that the depersonalization and the dehumanization associated with the high technology of conventional medicine are themselves inimical to the goal of health for all.

The problematic legacy of modern medicine and the contemporary medical crisis

Despite the impressive array of technological achievements mustered by contemporary medical science, there is a mordant irony in the fact that the health of the general population in most of the industrial world has not improved substantially during the present century. [1,2,3] Proponents of high-tech medical science have been inclined to defend the tradition on the ground that mortality rates have decreased markedly during the last 150 years. Closer inspection of this claim, however, reveals that the statistics on mortality are for several reasons *not* the best medical indicators of the level of public health. Mortality rates, after all, reflect a quantitative measure of health, not necessarily a qualitative one. The life of an individual could be considerably prolonged in a comatose state, for example, through the extraordinary means provided by the appropriate life-support apparatus. Such a scenario betrays that an increase in longevity need not be equivalent to an improvement in health. It is also instructive to note that the decrease in mortality rates during the last century reflected the decline of deaths of adults from infectious diseases and tuberculosis. [4, 5] Since 1900 the decline in mortality rates has resulted largely from the decline in infancy and early childhood previously attributable to infectious disease. [6] With the decline of infectious diseases, however, modern society has witnessed the proliferation of new epidemics or "diseases of civilization," as they have come to be called, whose death toll has in effect cancelled out the gains which would otherwise accrue from the further decline in infectious disease. [7, 8] Indeed, since the turn of the century, there has *not* been a substantial reduction in the rates of mortality for adults. Since 1900, in Australia, for example, the life span of 50-year-old male has at best been extended by only eight years. [9] This statistic is all the more contextualized when we see that males succumb more frequently to coronary heart disease and cerebrovascular disease than do women. What modest increase there has been in life expectancy over the past century admits of explanation by reference to the decline in deaths for infants and among the very young- as the statistics might at first glance suggest, to the lengthening of the overall lifespan. Indeed, there is evidence to show that the average life expectancy of males and females living in Counties in the United States has actually fallen. [10]

When all is said, even by the measure of mortality, we are not as a population healthier; we have simply substituted one form of disease for another. Tuberculosis, rheumatic fever, cholera, and polio have virtually disappeared from the industrialized world, but heart disease, emphysema, bronchitis, diabetes, and cancer have appeared in their place. In 2004 deaths resulting from cardiovascular disease accounted for 30 percent of all deaths worldwide, with an additional 13 percent of all deaths ascribed to cancer. In 1910, when William Olser delivered his lecture on angina pectoris to the Royal College Physicians of London, he asserted that coronary heart disease was a rare malady, afflicting only 20-25 per million in England and Wales. [11] It is now the leading cause of death in middle-aged men and women, and its overall incidence has soared from Osler's estimate of 20-25 per million [12] to one in every two men and one in every three women in 2001 in the United Kingdom. [13] The incidence of lung cancer worldwide has doubled since 1974 from 45 per 100,000 to 90 per 100,000 in 2000, accounting for 18 percent of all deaths attributed to cancer. [14] Both coronary artery disease and lung cancer are directly linked to smoking, thus it is of no surprise given the consumption of tobacco worldwide that cancer of the lung is the most common cause of death in men and women from industrialized nations. [15] In England and Wales the crude mortality rates of breast cancer has increased 12 percent between 1995 and 2004. [16]

Other signs of ill health among the general population are becoming more conspicuous and confirm the crisis in health care. It has been estimated, for example, that in excess of 86 million Americans, including one out of every three adult males, are afflicted with hypertension, one of the primary predisposing conditions causally associated with diseases of the heart and arterial system. [17] Slightly higher are the number of Americans who suffer from sleep-onset insomnia that now stands at approximately one third or 100 million of Americans, and another 46 million are besieged by the crippling effects of arthritis and rheumatism. Regular headaches are experienced by some 12 million Americans [18] and approximately 13 million children and adolescents and 67 million adult Americans, are estimated to be significantly outside their optimal weight range. [19] In a report by the Surgeon General from the United States National Public Health Service on Mental Health (1999) it was estimated that nearly 700,000 Americans were treated for alcoholism, while 15 percent of the population required some form of mental health services. [20]

Searching for instant relief from discomfort and stress, the population of the western world has taken to consuming utterly staggering quantities of prescription and nonprescription drugs. Aspirin, for example, is consumed at a rate of some 40 million pounds per year or 166 tablets annually per person. [21] Between 1990 and 2002 prescriptions written for prescription drugs such as Librium and Valium rose 25 percent, totaling 3, 340,000 prescriptions or 12 prescriptions per person per annum, [22] despite the fact that they all exhibit a high propensity for addiction and in some cases induce severe withdrawal symptoms. [23] While the statistics on the use of illegal drugs are more difficult to ascertain, it is clear that western society is rife with drug abuse, deleterious to health.

The social condition which signals the crisis in health care can also manifest themselves in subtle forms of threats to health. Consider the fact that when polio was at its peak, the death rate from that disease was approximately one twentieth as high as the death rate for males aged 15-24 which resulted from accidents. [24] Accidents combined with suicide and homicides, account for three out of every four male deaths in the 15-24 age category today. [25] Only three decades ago the *overall* death rate among this age group was 15 per cent lower, and in respect of the rate for violent deaths it was 40 per cent lower. [26] Bruckenwell expressed a sound intuition when he averred that we are in the midst of a crisis in health, to which the actions of young men have contributed significantly. [27]

So it comes that we have replaced the scourge of infectious disease, due primarily to poor hygiene and sanitation, with the chronic debilitating diseases of twentieth-century indulgences enshrined in the very structure of society. It is clear that the diseases and epidemics of modern civilization will not disappear through the genius and innovation of high-technology medicine, including skillful deployment of the surgeon's scalpel. Part of the difficulty is that what is required to promote the health of the community is not the high-technology intervention of the conventional medical kind to which our society has grown accustomed. Medical science can no more be justifiably praised for the elimination of contagious diseases than it can be condemned for its failure to contain and extirpate chronic and degenerative ones. In a special sense the pathology of disease lies deeply embedded in the psyche of the human race. We have established or tolerated the establishment of social institutions which ensure that we are not only environmentally assaulted, but alienated and dehumanized, sedentary and under exercised; even when overfed, we are more often than not poorly fed.

Consider, for example, the way in which we are constantly bombarded by commercials for soft drinks, candy products, and sweets of literally countless kinds, high fat and high salt foods, along with an almost endless barrage of processed foods. Capra reports one study in which four U.S. television stations in Chicago were analyzed to determine the role played by advertisements for food. [28] It was concluded that on weekdays over 70 percent, and on weekends over 85 per cent of the food commercials which appeared were negatively related to the advancement of community health. In another study it was concluded that each hour in the United States and Australia there are between 10 and 12 advertisements or 200 advertisements over a 20 hour period that are aimed at children, many of them advertising foods that are known, when consumed daily, to compromise human health. [29] For example, in 1997, in the United States, 7.3 billion dollars was spent on advertising children's breakfast cereals (792 million), candy and gum (765 million), soft drinks (549 million), and snack foods (330 million), yet in contrast to the exorbitant amount spent on advertising these products only 333 million dollars was spent on nutrition education. [30] Hence, nutrition education, utilized as a tool to improve health awareness was given less than four percent of the advertising expenditure than that of foods which are known to have negative health implications for humans, negative health implications that government organizations around the world are attempting to eradicate.

It is clear that excess sugar consumption is a nutritional culprit in most of the degenerative diseases peculiar to our society, including cardiovascular and cerebrovascular disease, the leading causes of death in western society. Our rich sugar diets are also associated with diseases such as diabetes, arthritis, obesity, and cancer. Nonetheless, average annual sugar consumption in the U.S. has increased by 28 percent since 1983, with sugar consumption per person estimated at 7280 tablespoons of refined sugar per year or 66 pounds of sugar per American. [31] This being so, it is no surprise to discover that approximately one-third of the entire American population is overweight. [32] This is no minor problem, as it is becoming increasingly evident that obesity is itself a disease and those individuals who are only 10 per cent overweight expose themselves to hormonal and immune-system deficiencies which in turn markedly increase their chances of acquiring any of the cadre of degenerative diseases known to modern civilization. [33] It has been estimated that of the 547,500 people who die of cancer in the U.S. every year, nearly 80 percent of the deaths predicted will be attributed to environmental factors including smoking and inadequate diet. [34] Once this point is appreciated, it is easier to understand that the resolution of the crisis in health care requires an approach to disease which is far more comprehensive than its analysis in bioreductionist and behaviorist terms permits. Contrary to the conventional wisdom, the fact is that the institution of professional medicine, no matter how technologically sophisticated, does not in itself have the power to make us healthy, and therefore it cannot be held fully responsible when, as a society, we are not healthier. If we are reflective and honest, it is clear that we have relinquished our responsibility for health to social institutions which have no genuine means to guarantee it. By making health professionals and the institutions they represent the custodians of health care, we diminish our own capacity to advance health on an individual and community basis.

Non-medical factors of health

In regard to the crisis in health care we are partly victims of our own ignorance and knowledge on the one hand and of our greed and indifference on the other. We perpetuate social mores and values which inspire lifestyles that are fundamentally unhealthy. The much-publicized tragedy of Love Canal is a case in point. [35] An abandoned trench in a residential area of Niagara Falls, New York, Love Canal was converted into a dumpsite for toxic waste. Over the course of years the chemical poisons from the Canal contaminated the surrounding bodies of water and eventually filtered into the gardens and yards of local residents. This process of chemical seepage led in turn to the generation of toxic fumes, a fact realized too late when it was discovered that their presence was associated with the disproportionately high rates of birth defects, respiratory ailments, kidney and liver damage, and a variety of forms of cancer exhibited by residents of the area. The extensive investigations which followed revealed that a significant portion of the American population are living on or in proximity to what have come to be called "toxic time bombs." In 1979 the U.S. Environmental Protection Agency produced statistics to show that of the staggeringly vast quantities of hazardous waste materials stored or buried in the *fifty thousand* known repositories for toxic waste across the U.S., only 7 percent can be said to have received the proper treatment necessary for their safe disposal. [36] The dimensions of the problem have become even more frightening for in 2005 the United States Environmental Protection Agency was shown to field 142 new chemical compounds per week, [37] and that the amount of hazardous waste had increased from ten to forty-one *million tons* during the past two decade. [38]

The medical profession has been unable to advance the overall health of the community for the simple reason that community health is the responsibility of the whole community, not just one institutional manifestation of it. It is also clear, moreover, that the orientation of conventional medicine has been towards "crisis medicine," i.e., the provision of medical treatment once illness and disease have struck. Two points should be stressed here. First, to equate advances in the technology of "crisis medicine" with advances in the level of community health is simply spurious. The treatment of disease is not the same as its eradication. Conventional medicine has long been preoccupied, as we observed in the previous chapter, with the *process* of disease, with the analysis, that is to say, of the biological mechanisms which define disease in structural terms. The eradication of disease lies in understanding its *origins* in a much wider sense. Consistent with the foregoing discussion it is evident, for example, that the relationship of the living organism to its environment is a salient factor in any comprehensive account of the origins of disease, the rectification of which may have more to do with *education* than with medical treatment of the signs or symptoms of disease.

Indeed, it is becoming increasingly clear that attempts to deal with disease, *simply* by introducing a form of treatment which remedies its organic signs (a bacteriological manifestation may itself be only a sign of disease) often prove to be only cosmetic. In failing to discern the sundry interfaces between the psychological and physical patterns of disease, and the influences of the environment upon them, conventional medical treatment may achieve little more than affecting a shift of the person's organically manifested response to, say, stress from one mode of disease or illness to another. The inability to establish a constructive dynamic of self-organization as a response to stress, that is to say, may result in any one of a variety of organic manifestations of disease. To cure a particular manifestation of the disease pattern (e.g., surgical intervention on a tumor) may well have its genesis untouched, and thus the treatment - though seemingly successful on one level - may have failed in making the person healthier at the deeper level. The removal of the tumor may in fact simply serve to reinforce and activate the very dynamics which stimulate the growth of another tumor or bring about another disease altogether, say, emphysema, as a way of compensating for the loss of the tumor.

The second point to be borne in mind is that, in regard to public health, the majority of the spectrum of diseases and illnesses, which plague mankind are resistant to the arsenal of techniques and medicines at the doctor's disposal. In a meticulous study drawing on three centuries of health statistics from England and Wales, McKeown has convincingly argued that only 10 percent of the improvement in mortality from infectious disease can be accounted for by the interventionist approach to health, including the use of antibiotics. [39] Speaking of illness in general, Dr. Herbert Benson of the Harvard Medical School has averred that at least three-quarters of the illnesses with which medicine is expected to deal with are either incurable in conventional terms or self-limiting, that is, capable of defining their own patterns of recovery. [40] The role of conventional medicine in securing public health is denied even more fervently by Ivan Illich, who states that beyond a certain level of intensity, institutional health care, no matter whether it takes the form of cure, prevention, or even environmental engineering, is bound to be counterproductive of health. [41] The greater the medical monopoly on health, the greater the encroachment on our liberty in respect of the management of our own bodies. By expropriating the power of individual self-reliance in favor of professional expertise, institutionalized medicine unwittingly decimates the potential resource of the entire population as the means of improving health. [42] The process of autonomous healing, so essential to the maintenance and advancement of health, is sacrificed in the name of professional competence. The rub is, as we shall see, that the goal of health for all remains as elusive to the professional expertise of the contemporary doctor as it did to purported powers of magic of the ancient practitioner.

Perhaps the most damning indictment of all, then, is contained in the charge that the crisis in health care is a result of our indifference to the continuation of those institutions of our creation that disempower us in regard to our bodies on the one hand and to our bond with nature on the other. We are thus brought full circle to the connection between health and virtue, between disease or illness and lifestyle. In essence we show that we value health by showing that we value ourselves, and our lifestyle is the social mirror of our values. Learning to value health and learning to value ourselves are two sides of the same coin. The crisis in health care is in part a crisis of the value of learning and also of the learning of value. This is why education is so crucial a factor in the advancement of community health and why autonomy is so crucial a factor in education. This is a theme to which we will revert in later chapters.

The prohibitive cost of health care and the problems of access to medical care

A time of crisis, however, is also a time of change, and conventional medicine is - as a result of growing dissatisfaction with a number of its aspects - in a state of transition. The Chinese have long been cognizant of the dynamics of crisis, and the Chinese term for "crisis," *wei-ji* represents the conjunction of two distinct characters, "danger" and "opportunity". [43] Both concepts apply to the current crisis in health care. There is danger of collapse, and there is opportunity for renewal. One danger which signals a particular direction of renewal is connected with the loss of credibility in regard to the cost-benefit analysis of conventional medicine. Illich, for instance, takes as the starting point of his examination the premise that conventional medicine is costly and ineffective. Let us see why.

The escalating costs of health care are undeniable. Between 1950 and 1965 the cost of health care in the U.S. increased from 10 to 40 billion dollars, from 4 to almost 6 percent of the gross national product (GNP). In 1965 the cost of a hospital bed was $40 per day; daily hospital costs in the U.S. now average in excess of $200. Between 1950 and 1977 the cost of health care accelerated at almost twice the pace of *all* other costs. The total health care cost in the U.S. for the fiscal year ending September 30, 1977 was 162.6 billion dollars, or 8.8 percent of the GNP, an average expenditure of $737 per person and an increase of 12 percent over the previous year. [44] However, despite the exorbitant costs of the past, when compared to the current health care costs of the United States they represent a minute portion of the costs now spent on health care. According to the United States Department of Health and Human Services, in 2005 the United States spent two trillion dollars on health care or 7,626 dollars per person, a sum which now exceeds 16 percent of the Gross Domestic Product. [45] In the early 1970s a House of Representatives subcommittee reported on the fact that in the late 1960s some 20-30 percent of American children were undergoing tonsillectomies and adenoidectomies, though no more than 2 to 3 percent of them could actually be regarded as appropriate candidates for these procedures. [46] As a consequence of these ill-advised surgical procedures, some 300 deaths resulted, and along with the estimated 15,000 operative and post-operative complications involved came equally unnecessary costs of 150 million dollars per year. In respect of other surgical procedures the subcommittee reported the loss of 11,900 lives resulting from 2.3 million unnecessary operations each year at a cost of 3.9 billion dollars. [47] In 2001 Null et. al wrote that these figures had risen considerably with an estimated 7.5 million unnecessary surgeries that resulted in 38,000 deaths at a cost of 122 billion dollars. [48] In the last two years, it is estimated that the cost of medical care in the United States has risen by 18.7 percent, in comparison to a 4.4 percent rise in the cost of living over the same period. [49] Along with these increases, the cost of health insurance has also escalated, and it has recently not been uncommon for Americans to bear annual increases of 50 to 100 percent in their health insurance premiums. [50]

The distribution of medical resources is in itself interesting given the claim that the continual increases in the costs of high-technology health care do not seem to have led to better health. In 2000, for example, more than 95 percent of U.S. health care resources were deployed in the service of disease treatment, less than 2.5 percent being used for research and prevention, and only a meager 0.5 percent spent on health education. In excess of 75 percent of the total health care budget was spent on treating illnesses such as cancer, stroke, and heart disease in their final stages. [51] The priorities expressed by past funding allocations have changed surprisingly little during the past two decades, though health costs have continued to escalate.

The myth of high-tech medicine

The first major challenge to the integrity of conventional medicine came in 1959 when Rene Dubos urged in his book *Mirage of Health* that the technological innovations of modern medicine, including the development of antibiotics, had far less to do with the improved health of the community than it might at first appear. [52] Amassing an impressive array of statistics in support of his claim, Dubos argued that the most significant changes in the health of the population derived from social, economic, and nutritional advances. Environmental factors not clinical care factors, were applauded as the primary determinants of the improved state of general public health. Better housing, for example, meant less overcrowding, thereby reducing the facility with which infectious disease was previously spread. Similarly, the provision of safe drinking water in conjunction with the treatment of sewerage dealt a forceful blow to infectious disease. Other environmental factors such as improved sanitary conditions and the effective disposal of garbage also had a beneficial impact upon the virulence and incidence of infectious disease. Heralded by some writers as the single most important factor in the decline of infectious disease, better nutrition has been acclaimed to assist host-resistance, as well as host-recovery. [53]

Indeed, by the time the etiology of infectious disease was sufficiently understood to develop and to administer vaccines, diseases such as cholera, typhoid fever, and dysentery had already been robbed of their virulence. In his presidential address in 1971 to the British Association for the advancement of Science, R. R. Porter confirmed that between 1860 and 1965 almost 90 percent of the total decline in mortality among children up to fifteen suffering from diphtheria, scarlet fever, measles, and whooping cough had occurred prior to the introduction of antibiotics and immunization on a systematic basis. [54] The virulence of tuberculosis had also declined markedly prior to the introduction of antibiotics. In 1812 the death rate from tuberculosis in New York was estimated to be higher than 700 per 10,000. When Koch first isolated and succeeded in culturing the bacillus in 1882, the death rate had dropped to 370 per 10,000. By the time the first sanatorium was opened in 1910 the rate had further declined to 180 per 10,000, until shortly after World War II it had slipped from second to eleventh place with a rate of 48 per 10,000. Still before antibiotics were used routinely, tuberculosis had flourished *and dwindled* outside the control of medical science. [55]

This is not to say that drug treatment has been entirely incidental in the decline of certain infectious disease. Syphilis and malaria were both quickly cured by chemotherapy. On the other hand, malaria has reappeared despite the continued use of anti-malarial drugs, largely because the use of pesticides was eventually superseded by the evolution of pesticide-resistant mosquitoes. Syphilis strains resistant to penicillin have also returned to remind medical science that the interlink between mores and medicine are of fundamental importance in understanding disease patterns.

Assessing the scope and limits of chemical and surgical intervention

Iatrogenic illness refers to those illnesses which result from professional medical treatment, and which could presumably have been avoided had such treatment not been administered. Ivan Illich has done much to consolidate and bring into bold relief studies concerning this category of physician- or hospital-caused injuries. He writes that "the pain, dysfunction, disability, and anguish resulting from technical medical intervention now rival the morbidity due to traffic and industrial accidents and even war-related activities, and make the impact of medicine one of the most rapidly spreading epidemics of our time."[56] Illich claimed that one out of every five persons entering a typical research hospital will acquire an iatrogenic disease. This figure is now estimated at one out of every three people, with iatrogenic disease now reported to be the third leading cause of disease in the United States.[57] Given that 2.8 billion outpatient prescriptions or 10 per person every year are written for Americans [58], it is perhaps unsurprising to find that one half of iatrogenic episodes arise from complications of drug therapy. [59] For instance, some patients are given the wrong drugs whilst others are given drugs which are contaminated. Some patients receive injections with improperly sterilized syringes, while others are given combinations of drugs which in their chemical reactions to each other prove to be harmful. The main problem here, however, is not simply one of negligence. Although the well-considered and circumspect use of drugs may have a role to play in health care, chemotherapy is an interventionist technique whose importance and use has been greatly exaggerated. As Mendelsohn has put it:

> "Unfortunately, doctors have seeded the entire population with these powerful drugs. Every year, from 8 to 10 million Americans go to the doctor when they have a cold. About ninety- five percent of them come away with a prescription - half of which are for antibiotics. . . . The doctor, once the agent of cure, has become the agent of disease. By *going too far* and diffusing the power of the extreme on the mean, Modern Medicine has weakened and corrupted even the management of extreme cases. The miracle I and other doctors were once proud to take part in has become a miracle of mayhem." [60]

While there has during the past decade been a growing awareness of the limitations of drugs therapy, the extent of the use and abuse of drugs in conventional medicine is still staggering. As a consequence of negative reactions to drugs, more than a 2.2 million people every year, or 3 to 5 percent of hospital admissions, are treated for drug complications. [61] It is also reported that a proportion of these patients will experience a second drug reaction during the course of their hospital stay. [62] The cost of health care associated with drug Mortality from toxicity in the United States is estimated at 12 billion dollars yearly, [63] and reflects the fact that a significant number of all hospital days are required to attend to patients suffering drug reactions. [64] Despite the growing use of street drugs, deaths attributed to medically prescribed drugs still exceed the number of deaths caused by the use of illegal drugs. It has been estimated that approximately 30,000 deaths per year are the consequence of adverse reactions to drugs prescribed by doctors. Serious reactions to drugs as common as penicillin, for example, occur at a rate of 6.5 per 100 adult admissions. [65] The anaphylactic shock which results from severe penicillin allergy is often more debilitating than the medical condition the penicillin was used to treat. Clammy skin, profuse sweating, fallen blood pressure, cardiovascular collapse, and even unconsciousness are just a few of the side-effects of acute reaction to penicillin. During the 1960s the drug tetracycline was administered so frequently that it came to be called the "housecall" antibiotic and a generation of children in America and elsewhere has suffered its adverse effects. In 1970 the U.S. Food and Drug Administration finally required that a warning be affixed to all packages of the drug, admonishing of the tendency of tetracycline to accumulate in bones and teeth. [66] One of the more visible side-effects of this chemical deposition has been to cause the permanent discoloration of developing teeth (i.e., stages of tooth development ranging from the last half of pregnancy to approximately eight years of age). Countless adults now bear their "tetracycline scars" on their teeth in shades of discolored enamel ranging from yellow to yellow-green to gray-brown.

Illich's study showed that one in every thirty cases of iatrogenic illness *leads to death* and that the frequency of reported accidents in hospitals exceeds the accident rates in all industries with the exceptions of mining and high-rise construction. [67, 68] Of all children admitted to hospitals, 25 percent will suffer an accident for which specific treatment will be required. [69,70] In a study of medical malpractice conducted by the United States Department of Health, Education, and Welfare, it is reported that 12 percent of all patients suffer compensable injuries while hospitalized, although only between 5 and 20 percent of these actually take legal action. [71] In a study by Bergman and Stamm on misdiagnosis, it was calculated that the number of children who suffer disability as a consequence of medical treatment for what turned out to be *cardiac nondisease* exceeds the number of children under effective treatment for genuine cardiac disease. [72]

In other cases it has been shown that specific forms of treatment actually exacerbate the specific condition they are intended to alleviate. The epidemic of asthma deaths in the mid-1960s provides a useful illustration. In England and Wales between 1959 and 1966 mortality due to asthma trebled in the age group 5-24 and increased seven-fold in the 10-14 age group. [73, 74] Up to this time mortality rates from this cause had remained relatively constant for more than a century. Although the epidemic was shared by Scotland, Ireland, Australia, and New Zealand, asthma mortality in Europe, Japan and North America remained virtually stable. Once it was ascertained that the prevalence of asthma was not on the increase, investigators hypothesized that the epidemic of asthma deaths could be associated with the new form of treatment whose introduction roughly coincided with the steady increase in mortality rates.

Evidence of the excessive use of pressurized aerosols containing bronchodilator drugs correlated with asthma patient deaths. Other investigations confirmed that the increase in asthma mortality correlated with the increased sales of aerosol bronchodilators, particularly those containing the drug isoprenaline. [75] Additional evidence in favor of the causal connection between the epidemic in asthma mortality and the excessive use of bronchodilator drugs came in 1968 when the sales of these aerosols were regulated in the United Kingdom by prescription. [76] Within a year asthma mortality rates declined and leveled off to almost pre-epidemic rates. Isoprenaline came under immediate suspicion since it was in any case the drug mainly used as a bronchodilator in the 1960s, though considerable debate ensured as to whether the fluorocarbon propellant could be cast as the true culprit. Although both isoprenaline and the fluorocarbon propellants were demonstrated to produce heart irregularities, it has more recently been shown that asthma mortality correlates particularly well with the sale of bronchiodilators capable of delivering up to five times the concentration of the normal spray of isoprenaline. It is estimated that in England and Wales the asthma epidemic claimed a total of 3,500 lives *in excess* of the expected rate over the same period calculated on the basis of the pre-epidemic rate in 1959-1960. [77] It has been remarked by Taylor that "even if some asthmatics were saved by medical treatment, more were lost."[78, 79]

The use of other medically prescribed drugs has led to the increased risk of other diseases worse than the ones that they are designed to treat. Reserpine, for example is one of the drugs which has been used to control high blood pressure. Despite the fact that studies undertaken in the mid-70s have established that reserpine triples the risk of breast cancer, already ranked as the number-one cause of death in women, it is still prescribed. There are now indications that insulin, heralded as one of the miracles of modern medicine, is implicated as one of the causes of diabetic blindness. [80] Investigations undertaken in the 1970s revealed that daughters of women treated with a synthetic oestrogen, Diethylstilbestrol (DES), during the early stages of pregnancy for the purported prevention of miscarriage are developing vaginal cancer at an alarmingly high rate. It has also been confirmed more recently that an alarmingly high incidence of genital malformation can be correlated with the male offspring of women treated with DES, not to mention that the cancer mortality rate of the women themselves is also statistically significant. Studies of DES have since established that it does not prevent miscarriage; indeed, it is in fact currently used as a "morning-after" contraceptive pill and in some cases to dry up milk. In the case of DES it is particularly ironic that here we have a drug that not only caused vaginal cancer and other abnormalities, but did not even work for the purpose for which it was originally administered. [81]

DES is not the only hormone which - despite detrimental side-effects - doctors prescribe for women. While it is to be admitted that there has in recent years been a greater awareness of the drug-associated victimization of patients to which we have been alluding, the fact that some 27 percent of women in the United States alone are under prescription for the birth control pill [82] or menopausal estrogens gives cause for reflection. Concern about the side-effects of the pill led the U.S. Food and Drug Administration to issue a warning bulletin to doctors in 1975 exhorting that women beyond the age of forty be taken off the Pill and provided other means of contraception. The first admonition was followed by a second from the FDA in 1977 requiring the provision of a warning brochure stressing the inordinately high risk of cardiovascular disease among women over forty taking the Pill. [83] The mortality risk from cardiovascular disease for women over forty taking the Pill is increased by a *factor* of five; for women between the ages of thirty to forty the risk of dying from a heart attack is multiplied by a factor of three. Increased risk of cardiovascular disease is not the only health hazard associated with the Pill. The risk of high blood pressure is six times greater for women taking the Pill than for those who are not. Women taking the Pill run a risk of thromboembolism which is more than five times that for women not taking it and the risk of stroke is four times greater. [84, 85] Other health risks associated with the Pill are liver tumors, headaches, depression, and cancer. [86]

Similarly, anti-hypertension drugs have in recent years soared in popularity as an easy way to lower blood pressure. Although medical journals carry advertisements for drugs intended to counteract the adverse effects of anti-hypertension drugs, sufficient awareness of their dangers seems decidedly *not* to be reflected by the astronomical number of medical prescriptions still written for them. Among the multitude of side effects associated with high blood pressure drugs are rash, hives, sensitivity to light, vertigo, muscle cramps, weakness, inflammation of the blood vessels, joint aches, muscle spasms, nausea, psychological disorientation, reduced libido, and impotency (affecting women as well as men). [87]

Medical intervention utilizing the tools of high technology has also given rise to its own peculiar forms of iatrogenic diseases. Between the years 1942 and 1954 the problem of retrolental fibroplasias, disease of the eye leading to blindness, came to figure prominently in the management of premature infants in the United States. Despite being possessed of some of the most advanced medical technology available, hospital nurseries especially equipped to accommodate premature babies were finding that around *ninety percent* of all low-weight infants suffered either partial or total blindness. Indeed by 1954 retrolental fibroplasias ranked *first* in the United States among the causes of blindness in children. [88] Investigations eventually showed that the increasing incidence of the disease paralleled the introduction of plastic incubators into which high concentrations of oxygen were pumped to the premature infants on the assumption that oxygen therapy was beneficial, an assumption which, during the time high-concentration oxygen therapy was used, was in fact untested. Oxygen therapy did make the babies look pink, but definitive evidence was provided in 1954 by Lanman et al. that it also made them go blind. [89]

Another example of the extent to which high-technology medicine can be debilitating is amply demonstrated by the controversy surrounding coronary arteriography, a test technique whereby a dye is injected into the coronary arteries by way of a small catheter threaded from one of the blood vessels in the limbs and back towards the heart. The technique is designed to assist in the diagnosis and evaluation of coronary heart disease by providing an outline of the interior of the coronary arteries through the medium of the passage of the dye which is visible on X-ray film. In support of the procedure, mortality rates of 0.1 percent or one per thousand are cited to indicate the technique to be a relatively innocuous one. Taylor has commented, however, that the statistics belie the true state of affairs. The mortality rate of one per thousand is accurate, he says, if the statistical analysis is restricted to results of the procedure deriving from only "very competent" and "experienced" units which perform it. Surveys of the technique which reflect a regional and more comprehensive base reveal quite different statistics. When the review of the more comprehensive practice of coronary arteriography was carried out, it showed that the mortality rates was not one per thousand, but virtually one in every hundred, ten times the rate regarded as innocuous. The death rate for patients undergoing the procedure in some institutions was as high as 8 percent, the incidence of cardiac arrest during the procedure, in respect of which defibrillation was required to resuscitate the heart, ranged from 1 - 10 percent. Some studies report that in addition to the threat of mortality, serious complications resulting from coronary arteriography are of the order of 1.5 per cent. [90]

X-rays represent another dimension of high-technology medicine whose unbridled use has led to untold iatrogenic illness and disease. Mendlesohn reports that thyroid lesions, a considerable number of which are proving to be cancerous, "are turning up by the thousands in people who were exposed to head, neck, and upper chest radiation twenty to thirty years ago." [91] The amount of radiation required to cause thyroid cancer, he asserts, is "less that that produced by ten lite-wing dental X-rays." [92] It is sobering to hear that every year some 4,000 people die from radioactive dental and medical interventionist techniques, and there are those who urge that the estimate is conservative. [93] The use of X-rays to diagnose and assess the female breast is - despite the iatrogenic problems associated with them - widely recommended as an effective means of detecting breast cancer in its early stages. Setting aside the fact that studies have shown that disagreement among radiologists is considerable in respect of their interpretation of the same film, it is even more distressing to find that other studies reporting that mammography will in fact cause more breast cancer than it will detect and that the number of deaths from breast cancer caused by mammography may in fact "balance the number of patients who may be cured by early diagnosis and treatment of the naturally occurring disease. [94] Putting aside the cancer-causing effects of mammography, the efficacy of the procedure in correctly diagnosing cancer can be questioned. At one Australian teaching hospital between 1979 and 1988, 218 women attended for mammography, in 95 of which cases the mammogram failed to detect breast cancer. [95] For 47 of these, delayed treatment had tragic results. [96, 97]

Specific iatrogenic diseases resulting from surgical intervention are astronomical in number and kind. Complications arise from lack of surgical expertise, the degree of difficulty involved in performing the surgery, the unique constitution of the patient, anaesthetic accidents, lacerations of large blood vessels, and misplace ligatures disrupting nerve responses and blood flow.

Taylor reports that an untold variety of surgical instruments, swabs, etc. have been left and sutured to cause serious infection. Even the talc commonly used by surgeons to lubricate their hands so that their surgical gloves can be more easily fitted is now known to cause inflammatory reactions in patients on whom they operate. Uncontrollable internal bleeding, shock, coma, and death are not uncommon side effects of surgical intervention. [98]

The crisis of depersonalization in contemporary western medicine and the problem of 'professional affective detachment'

From even our brief discussion of iatrogenic disease it should be clear that the side effects resulting from drug, instrumental, and surgical intervention are almost limitless. There is, however, another aspect of iatrogenesis which is more subtle than the obvious intrusions of a physical kind to which we have been referring. The bioreductionist philosophy which underpins conventional medical science has given rise to a highly technological form of health care which is by its very nature debilitating and subversive of the autonomous mechanisms by virtue of which self-healing and self -care take place. Despite the fascination of high-technology medicine, many health practitioners have long been aware of an element in the healing process which is determinative of the body's reaction to illness, of its capacity to resist it, to transform it, and to overcome it. This element of mind or indomitable spirit, if one prefers, is not amenable to bioreductionists' tests or to microscopic *analysis.*

In part the recent discipline of *psychosomatic medicine* represents an important development away from bioreductionism in the hope of explicating the nature of the mind-body interface in medically relevant ways. Out of psychosomatic medicine has evolved the even newer discipline of *phychoimmunology,* founded largely on the research of the Russian E. A. Korneva and followed by the work of George Solomon and Alfred Amkraut, which recognized the importance of the subtle but specific interplay between the mind and the immune system. The work of Robert Ader has reinforced this movement, though his particular emphasis upon the role of the central nervous system in the disease process led to the word "neuro" being inserted into the name given by Solomon to his new discipline; phychoimmunology thus became *psychoneuroimmunology* or PNI. [99] Reactions to PNI research from more traditional quarters of medicine have on occasion been openly hostile, so much so that Solomon left PNI research because, as he put it, "no one would listen." [100]

One aspect of bioreductionist medicine which has in fact been disruptive of the integrity of the mind-body interface and thus *covertly iatrogenic* in respect of the process of healing, has been its tendency to depersonalize the fundamentally social aspects of heath care by the progressive substitution of technological innovation for the phenomenon of human interchange. This aspect of the degradation of health is seldom, if ever, classified as iatrogenic, and though we believe a more perspicacious picture of the crisis in health care emerges from doing so. To endeavor to isolate a particular technological development as *the first* piece of technology which served to initiate the depersonalization process in health care would doubtless be fatuous. There seems to be a measure of consensus among historians of medicine, however, that the development of the stethoscope was one of the developments which set the trend in motion. It was in 1819 that Rene Laennec introduced the technique of *Auscultation* in which medical diagnosis could be made by listening to the internal sounds of the human body. Laennec's invention of the stethoscope was hailed as affording doctors non-surgical access into hitherto inaccessible domains of the body. Since then, the use of the stethoscope has become one of the basic rituals of modern medicine, though some commentators such as Mendlesohn have opined that it does more harm than good, passing contagion from patient to patient. [101] More pertinent to our notion of "iatrogenesis through depersonalization," however, is the way in which the technology of the stethoscope has transformed ineradicably the person and intimate character of the physical examination. The traditional and intimate practice of the physician having to place an ear to the patient's chest was eliminated in favor of the more detached method of examination afforded by the stethoscope. In essence the human and personal touch was replaced by the impersonal touch of technology. As Lewis Thomas writes in his engaging book, *The Youngest Science*:

> "Touching with the naked ear was one of the great advances in the history of medicine. Once it was learned that the heart and lungs made sounds of their own, and that the sounds were sometimes useful for diagnosis, physicians placed an ear over the heart, and over areas on the front and back of the chest, and listened. It is hard to imagine a friendlier human gesture, a more intimate signal of personal concern and affection, than the close-bowed head affixed to the skin". [102]

By the mid -1880's the doctor's arsenal of diagnostic devices had grown considerable and included the ophthalmoscope (to facilitate the examination of the eyes), the otoscope (for examining ears), and the laryngoscope (for assessment of the throat). During the course of the nineteenth and twentieth century's, the proliferation of medical technology such as the diagnostic tools and instruments enumerated in the first chapter encouraged an approach in which the patient was regarded progressively as an *object* of study – as an impersonal body or machine on which clinical tests could be performed and diagnostic instruments used. With the introduction of separate diagnostic tests for specific illnesses, the collection of data and relevant statistics took on a new importance and shifted the doctor's attention from the patient to the patient's disease and from the patient's disease to the concatenation of data and statistics presumed to quantify and objectively to represent it. The role of the patient's subjective experience of illness was thus displaced as the locus of medical attention in favor of the technological interpretation of it. As the complexity of medical technology increased, the demands on doctors in respect of technological expertise also increased. With the advent of X-rays, CAT scanners, the electrocardiogram, the electroencephalagram, blood tests, and the like, doctors were required to know not only about the etiology of disease, but about the sundry interpretations of the amalgam of medical data upon which the treatment of disease had been made to depend. As the medical world came to rely progressively upon the technological innovations designed to diagnose, assess, and cure disease, the role of the patient in the process of healing was in consequence progressively devalued.

Regardless of the subtlety of individual differences in disease manifestation, the bioreductionist model encouraged a taxonomy of disease in which patients were fitted to diseases amenable of classification. Patients have thus come to be regarded as "disease-specimens," and labeled according to their diseases. The institutional expression of this form of depersonalization and dehumanization has shown itself in the tendency of doctors and staff to *identify* people by reference to the diseases from which they suffer. One thus hears nonliteral metaphors such as the "*cholecystectomy* in bed four" or the "*cardiovascular* in ward 2" used to describe *persons* who are otherwise identifiable by their names. Treating a patient, on this orientation, thereby amounts to little more than "something that is done *to* the patient," not something that we help patients to do for themselves.

Technological iatrogenesis, then, is not merely a matter of the disease and illness caused as a direct result of technological intervention into the body. By depersonalizing the process of healing, high-technology medicine proliferates disease and illness unwittingly by disrupting and stifling the very mechanisms for healing in respect of which the patient and doctor alike are *personally* involved. High-technology medicine has, we suggest, been particularly abusive of the human personality, for it covertly denies the nonquantifiable aspects of the interplay between mind and body which define a personality as healthy or unhealthy. The bioreductionist tradition in medicine has, when all is said, bequeathed to posterity a self-perpetuating technology whose prohibitive cost may on the one hand outweigh its benefits to health, and on the other, ensure that those benefits are of such a kind that they belie the deeper source of the illnesses of which they treat.

The pervasive influence of iatrogenic illness is not as easily eliminated as some commentators - even those critical of bioreductionism - suggest. The problem is not *simply* a matter of the excessive or inappropriate use of technological developments in respect of which drugs, medical instrumentation, and surgery all figure prominently. We have seen, for example, that the problems associated with the over-prescription of antibiotics have not - contrary to all expectations - served to ensure that doctors would be more circumspect in their prescription of hormones, of anti-hypertension drugs, and more recently of anti-arthritic drugs such as Butazolidin alka, Motrin, Indocin, Naprosyn, Nalfon, Tolectin, all of which have now exhibited side-effects sufficiently potent to rival the menace to public health created by the drug epidemics which preceded them.

One reason for the persistent presence of iatrogenic illness and the difficulty involved in trying to eliminate it derives from the fact that bioreductionist medicine is by its very nature interventionist. Given the dominance of the bioreductionist concept of disease (i.e., that every disease or infection is caused by a specific microorganism), the orientation of health care will be directed to discovering new ways of making appropriate determinations concerning which microorganisms relate causally with which diseases. The battle against disease will thus be fought at the microscopic level, and technological intervention represents the mechanist way of fighting it. Drugs, technological devices, and surgery are thus part and parcel of the reductio-mechanist medical model. They are not, in essence, controlled—they are controlling. As Mendelsohn puts it:

> "Of course, if drugs were merely products of medical *science,* dealing with them would be a matter of science, rationality and common sense. But drugs aren't merely scientific—they're *sacred.* Like the communion wafer which Catholics receive on the tongue, drugs are the communion wafers of Modern Medicine. When you rake a drug, you're communing with one of the mysteries of the Church: the fact that the doctor can alter your inward and outward state if you have the faith to take the drug." [103]

It is misleading to suggest that iatrogenic disease can be prevented as long as the use of drugs, surgery, and technological devices is not excessive, for the microscopic or molecular penetration of the body presupposed by the bioreductionist model is, by virtue of its depth of intervention, necessarily *excessive.* Lest we be misunderstood, this is not to say that such techniques are never appropriate—it is rather to say that iatrogenesis is an endemic feature of bioreductionist medicine, not one of its peripheral accoutrements or accidental byproducts. The key to the control of iatrogenesis lies in challenging the philosophical foundations of the bioreductionist model, not in trying independently to regulate the use of medical techniques which are in a much deeper sense themselves regulated by the model.

Summary

It has been our purpose in this chapter to show that conventional medicine is in a state of crisis and of transition. We have seen that the problems confronting western medicine relate to a crisis of costs, a crisis of health care, and a crisis of philosophical direction and orientation. Although during the past century substantial reductions in death and disability from infectious disease have occurred, modern medicine has been unable to stem the rising tide of chronic and degenerative diseases which now plague contemporary society as the prime agents of morbidity and mortality. Infectious disease has been replaced by cardiovascular disease, cerebrovascular disease, and cancer, all of which appear to demand more of technological medicine than it is capable of delivering. In the name of modern medicine we have spent progressively more money to treat diseases which by their very nature seem progressively less amenable to conventional treatment.

Increasingly, the annals of medicine are reporting the crippling iatrogenic effects of drugs, diagnostic tests, high-tech treatments, and surgical interventions previously presumed to be harmless or relatively innocuous. In this connection our aim was to show that more high-technology medicine does not necessarily amount to "better" medicine, and certainly not to better health care. The assumption that 'more is better' constitutes what we have called the "technological fallacy," and it is a fallacy for the following reason. That the side-effects of technological intervention can be eradicated by the development of even more sophisticated and powerful innovations of a technological kind misses the point that it is not just a *particular* aspect of technology which is the problem, but the *level and nature of technological intervention itself* which needs reconceptualization. The ever-expanding reliance upon high-tech medical techniques of an interventionist kind is motivated by a whole philosophy of nature in which the human organism is a machine—albeit a highly complicated one—whose 'essence' can be understood by breaking down the whole into its most fundamental material parts. In challenging the dominance of "medical technologization," our deeper intention is to challenge the philosophical assumptions upon which it rests.

Appreciation of the interplay between the technologization of medicine and the interventionist and reductionist philosophy which undergirds it makes it easier to see why we have introduced "iatrogenesis through depersonalization" as a category of iatrogenic disease. If the etiology of disease is reduced to its seat in structural or organic dysfunctions, then the interaction between the psyche and the immune system, for example, can easily be neglected. Our emphasis on iatrogenesis which results from the depersonalizing effects of technological medicine in its reductionist mode is thus intended to redress the imbalance arising from this neglect.

CHAPTER 3

Taking our blinkers off: Tapping the potential for health through wholism

Disenchantment with the current theory and practice of medicine has, we have seen, led to renewed interest, almost of a Socratic kind, concerning the role which education plays in the maintenance of public health and the prevention of disease. We also observe that health education which is conceived on the limited perspective of the bioreductionist model is bound to be inadequate, representing an incomplete approach to health care. Although there has, outside the traditional medical community and to a lesser extent within it, been a certain receptivity to the notion of wholistic health, it is clear that the philosophical foundations which define and direct its coherent implementation give a whole new sense to the conventional concepts of health and disease.

In truth, wholistic medicine is not yet a well-defined discipline. Encompassing a vast array of unorthodox therapies such as reflexology, homeopathy, chelation therapy, iridology, acupuncture, Rolfing, therapeutic touch, color therapy, Alexander technique, human aura therapy, crystal and psychic therapy, wholism is as much a social and philosophical movement as it is a distinctive approach to medicine. This is an extremely important point for it implies that one could accept the basic philosophy of wholism without necessarily endorsing the whole spectrum of therapeutic techniques which claim to be expressions of it. The failure to make this distinction is the cause of considerable confusion, as attested by the unbridled invective against wholistic medicine by Stalker and Glymour in their book, *Examining Wholistic Medicine.* Charging that the specific alternative therapies offered by wholistic medicine are either unproven or palpably false, they mistakenly conclude "that the science of wholistic medicine is bogus; that the philosophical views championed by the movement are incoherent, uninformed, and unintelligent; and that most wholistic therapies are crank in the usual sense of that word: they lack any sound scientific basis." [1, 2] Threatened by the force of wholistic medicine as a *social* movement, their wholesale rejection of it as a *philosophical* alternative to conventional medicine is, as we note, gratuitous.

It is clear, for example, that the wholistic approach to health denies that disease can be explained satisfactorily *via* its reduction to the particular micro-organisms which, in the reductionist-mechanist paradigm, have come to be associated with it. It is also evident, on the wholistic view, that every living organism is an integrated whole, the understanding of which is lost in the reduction of the whole to basic properties of which it is composed. Since the biological mechanisms with which reductionist medicine concerns itself are - according to the wholistic model - seldom, if ever, the exclusive cause of illness and disease, the genuine eradication of illness and disease will seldom if ever depend simply upon interventionist techniques, no matter how sophisticated, which proscribe the orientation to health care in reductionist terms. This may be so, but philosophically we need to know why it is so.

Conventional health care on the bioreductionist model amounts to little more than "disease care." The wholistic approach, on the other hand, repudiates the notion that health can be properly understood as the absence of disease. Stressing the multidimensional character of living organisms and the essential interdependence between the state of a being and the biological, psychological, sociocultural, and environmental factors which impinge upon health and disease, the wholistic approach presupposes a philosophical commitment to the "systems view of life" which itself needs to be made explicit. If primary health care is to encompass the wholistic orientation to health, it must be capable of expressing through the process of "educating for health" the philosophical foundations upon which its theory and practice rests. In the present chapter we have therefore set ourselves the task of providing at least a tolerably coherent account of the concepts of health and disease which derive from the wholistic framework enunciated. In the context of this framework we will show that health is a process of dynamic adaptation of the organism to the environment. This being so, the way in which, as a culture, we relate ourselves to nature on the one hand and shape nature on the other has unrecognized health consequences of enormous import. The paradox is that in restructuring nature to facilitate the process of our own adjustment to it, we have unwittingly transformed the environment in ways which have made the process of adaptation more difficult, and in some cases, impossible. The view of health we propose thus entails an epistemology of ecology, part of which we have rehearsed in the previous chapter. We contend that this profoundly ecological and psychosocial view of health marks the boundaries of the new frontiers of health education. The virtue of this approach lies not so much in resurrecting the ancient wisdom of the past, either in its religious or scientific expressions, as in consolidating and synthesizing into a new vision of reality the philosophical components worth salvaging in both. Let us defer these proceedings no further.

Seeking coherence and avoiding 'wholistic quackery'

Although the use of the term "holism" has become increasingly fashionable, its precise meaning seems to have become increasingly obscure. "Holistic" is all too often employed as a covering concept for any of the arcane, exotic, or unconventional forms of healing. Alternative forms of medicine, for example, are often designated as being "wholistic" simply by virtue of being unconventional or alternative. [3] Some unconventional practitioners call themselves "wholistic healers" and utilize an entire collection of unconventional therapies which have little more *in common* philosophically than that they are *unconventional.* [4] Wholism is not to be equated with *eclecticism*, for eclecticism is not in itself a philosophical description of healing practices. Similarly, other therapies claim to be wholistic by virtue of their rejection of the scientific basis of modern medicine, while others proclaim the cause of wholistic health in the name of mind, body, and spirit, though the philosophical connections among these components and the forms of treatment to which they give rise remain obscure and heuristically otiose.[5] Other writers sometimes speak of "wholistic medicine" or "wholistic health," as if they were referring to a new and distinct discipline of medicine with its own peculiar body of knowledge amendable to investigation and study as one might investigate and study the accumulated wisdom of anatomy or physiology. All these definitions are, we believe, even when they contain an element of truth, misleading and vague.

The etymology of the term "wholism" offers some insight into a more substantial formulation of its lucid use. "Wholism" derives from the Indo-European root word *kailo,* which literally meant "intact," "uninjured," and "whole." Over time the root word *kailo* gave rise to a family constellation or words and concepts in different languages, including the Old English word *hale,* whose associations range from "holy" to "whole" to "heal" to "health," to name only a few. It would seem, nonetheless, that in its etymological origins the term "wholism" refers to a state or quality of being in which being *whole* (e.g., integrated or balanced) was to be associated with *health* and *healing.* [6]

It is this sense of the word that we wish to preserve in the use we will make of it. Wholism in health thus refers not to a body of knowledge as such or to a collection of therapies, but to a philosophical approach or methodological strategy whereby the issues of health and disease are viewed as features of the complex interplay between the *whole* person and the *total* environment. Let us try to clarify this.

As far as we can discern, the word "wholistic" was - despite the ancient origins of the basic concepts underpinning it - first coined in 1926 by Jan Christian Smuts. [7] In his book titled *Holism and Evolution,* Smuts employed the term "holism" to signify the teleological disposition of evolution. Biological organisms, he urged, are possessed of an innate capacity for self-maintenance and internal regulation, functioning constantly to correct imbalances which result from the particular interface between the particular organism and the environment. The tendency to self-healing characterized for Smuts the wholistic tendency or teleology of nature in its evolutionary manifestation.

The *wholistic* or organismic approach - contrary to the conventional wisdom - has in fact quite respectable scientific origins, though it has admittedly been dominated and suppressed by the bioreductionist one. [8, 9] In the 1930s Ludwig von Bertalanffy introduced Wholism as a conceptual component within General Systems Theory, and it is perhaps here that the concept of wholism received its most comprehensive development within conventional science. [10] Wholism has also been associated with other distinguished scholars of science such as J. B. S. Haldane, A. N. Whitehead, F. S. C. Northrop, Abraham Maslow, Paul Weiss, Rene Dubos and Joshua Freeman to name a few. [11]

As we conceive it, wholism affords a conceptual alternative to the reductionist paradigm which has long dominated the scientific approach to medicine. One way in which it does this is to force the reconceptualization of the fundamental concepts of health and disease in a way that allows for a philosophical synthesis of the contemporary eclecticism perpetrated in its name.

Building foundations for the edifice of wholism in health

Changes in the concepts of health and disease, as we observed in Chapter 1, have not occurred in accordance with a continuous and orderly process of evolution. As Dubos indicates, transformations of medical theory reflect "the prevailing view of man's nature and his relation to the cosmos." [12] Disease has thus been explicated variously by reference to demons, gods, sin, germs, and genetics. The "ontological doctrine," as Dubos calls it, refers to the doctrine of specific etiology or the view, as we saw earlier, that disease refers to specific entities independent of the individual's personality, physical and mental constitution, and even lifestyle.[13, 14] By conceptualizing disease as a micro-organism or germ external to the body which somehow gets into it, we implicitly relinquish responsibility for the infirmity with which we are afflicted. The mode of projection is betrayed in our vocabulary. The patient is, for example, prone to say, "I caught a cold" or "Something I ate made me sick," or, in the metaphorical language of constant *battle* against disease, "He was attacked by polio" or "She was overcome by flu." Disease is conceived as something apart from ourselves, as something that happens to us, and thus by implication as something over which the patient has little control. [15] In Chapter 1 we observed the extent to which this view of disease has been fostered by the reductionist medical model.

Causality and disease specificity are, to paraphrase Dubos, much less common in the clinical situation than in the confines of the laboratory. He points out that few pathological states can be represented by clinical pictures amenable to classification as biological entities. He writes:

> What the patient experiences and what the physician observes constitute generally a confusing variety of symptoms and lesions rather than a well-defined entity. In most cases, a syndrome such as anemia, cardiac insufficiency, gastric disturbance, and depression is more in evidence than the unique pathological manifestation of a specific etiological agent. Furthermore, each noxious agent can express itself by a great variety of pathological states. The phthisis studied by Laennec had little in common with the primary infection that is now the most common form of tuberculosis in our communities; yet both are caused by tubercle bacilli of the same virulence. [16]

Acknowledgement of causal anomalies such as these have made it easier to appreciate that disease patterns and manifestations are conditioned not so much by causative agents in the form of biological entities as by the responses of the organism as a whole in its dynamic interaction with them. Nor is the specific nature of such responses easily stereotyped either for groups of individuals or for the same individual at different times. It is now well-known, for example, that the adrenal and other hormones profoundly influence the immune and other responses to pathogenic agents. It is also known, moreover, that psychological factors such as the symbolic interpretation that the mind attaches to the context in which the etiological agent is presented and to the causative agent itself in turn conditions the salient patterns of secretion exhibited by these hormones. Disease can no more be comprehended through its correspondence to isolated biological entities than the function of an internal organ be understood without reference to the other organs and processes in respect of which it functions as an integrated structure. This recognition brings us to the *systems view of health and disease.*

The network concept of 'Systems Theory' and its implications for wholistic modeling of well-being

The gradual shift which marks the transition from the bioreductionist model of disease to the systems view has not been continuous and is not yet complete. Bioreductionism still constitutes the dominant philosophical disposition of medical theory and practice, but there is a new awareness of its limitations and deficiencies, as we have seen in the foregoing chapters. It has only been in recent years, however, that the conventional approach to health care in general has been challenged by disputing the assumptions which underpin it. Up to the time of the Second World War, for example, health was standardly defined as the absence of disease, and conversely, disease was defined as the absence of health. Indeed, for the most part the application of both concepts was restricted to descriptions signifying a purely physical state of well-being, with virtually no consideration being given to the array of emotional, social, and environmental factors affecting health. In 1946 the constitution of the World Health Organization was thought to be a*vant-garde* for defining health as "a state of complete physical, mental, and social well-being and merely the absence of disease or infirmity." [17]

This definition received a mixed reaction from the community of scholars. It has been commended by some writers and renounced by others. It has been applauded, as one might expect, for having expanded the concept of health to include aspects which in the standard definition have consistently been excluded. It has also been criticized for being hopelessly unrealistic. One such critic was Callahan, who writes unabashedly: "it is doubtful that there ever was, or ever will be more than a transient state of 'complete physical, mental and social well-being' for individuals or societies; that's not the way life is or could be."[18] Not only did he condemn the definition for being too ambitious to be possible of achievement, but he urged that a deeper danger for those who endorse it lay in encouraging unrealistic expectations or a "false consciousness" of the goal of health. [19] His polemic continues: "The demands which the word 'complete' entail set the stage for the worst false consciousness of all: the demand that life delivers perfection. Practically speaking, this demand had led in the field of health to constant escalation and requirement, never ending, never satisfied." [20] Even the general idea of trying to provide a precise definition of health has not always been met with optimism. In 1973 Seigel, for instance, enumerated a few of the problems confronting those who seek to define health. He suggests that the definition of health constitutes a value judgment, and refers to a personal and highly subjective state.[21] It is an abstraction without objective reference, and health is a relative concept which is culturally determined.[22, 23]

In an attempt to accommodate the concept of health as it reflects on the one hand the organized complexity of the diverse organic functions which constitute the integrated expression of the living organism and, on the other, the interface between the organism and the environment, the systems view of life was adapted to the medical and health care framework. [24] Although the systems approach has been applied in the area of health care management, the basic notion of extending it as a scheme for understanding health and disease has been surprisingly limited. This is an approach we favor, and following the work of Laszlo [25], which derives largely from the pioneering study mentioned earlier of Ludwig von Bertallanfy on general systems theory, we will elaborate a few fundamental concepts and then consider their application to the wholistic understanding of health and disease.

The term "system" refers to an organized set of components whose peculiar pattern of integration contributes to an indivisible whole or complex unit. Within the integrated whole are any of a number of interconnected parts whose peculiar relationships contribute to the character of the whole of which they are parts. The parts can remain the same, in other words, but if their organizational patterns are altered, the character of the whole is also altered. Conversely, any of the multifarious parts of a system could be replaced, even by different parts, and if the parts are not too dissimilar, the overall organization and logical integrity of the system will remain the same. Every organism, ranging from the enormous complexity of the human organism to the simplest bacterium, is regarded as an integrated whole and thus as "systemic." The relationship between parts and wholes is not circumscribed unidirectionally. The heart, for example, could be regarded as a system in itself with cellular components whose peculiar interrelationships define the integrity of the whole or, as we have already indicated, as a component part in the integrated whole whose boundaries are the entire living organism. In the same way, the living organism can be regarded as an integrated whole in itself or as a component part in a more comprehensive set of interrelationships which define other integrated wholes.

The term "hierarchy" refers to the classification which results when systems are ranked or organized in order of increasing complexity. Atoms could thus be regarded as subcomponents of molecules, and molecules as subcomponents of cells, extending the ranking relation from cells to tissues, from tissues to organs, and so on. The individual can be regarded as a whole or as a component, say, in a family, and similarly, a family can be regarded as a whole in itself or as a component in a community. "Higher-level system" is an expression which thus refers to the level of complexity in respect of the relationship ranking between systems. For a particular purpose the system chosen as the point of departure for the resolution of a problem will depend upon the particular problem, not the intrinsic level of complexity of the system. Certain aspects of liver disease, for example, might best be illuminated by reference to "tissue" as the primary system of analysis, whereas correlations between liver disease and drinking patterns might be explicated by reference to a higher-level system.

Although the concept of "hierarchy" reveals that such things as cells are made up of molecules, it does not tell us why molecules in a particular pattern constitute the integrated whole we define as a cell and why other collections of molecules do not. This is where the concept of "information flow" enters into general systems theory.

"Information" is defined broadly as that element which has the potential to re-order the activities of the components within the system. "Transaction" is the name given to the simultaneous and mutually interdependent activities which obtain among the multiple components of the system. A particular "flow of information" will determine this transaction, shaping the organizational patterns in ways which determine whether molecules are constituted as cells or as something else. The form commonly taken by the flow of information is known as a "feedback loop," implying that the logical relation which governs the organization of subcomponents is such that component A influences component B, but the altered state of B now feeds back to change the state of A. Regulation of the system of feedback is thought to be of two kinds, "negative" and "positive."[26] Negative feedback is designed to keep the system in homeostatic balance. Each of the subcomponent systems has a certain degree of latitude in respect of its activity, but beyond certain limits it jeopardizes the integrity of the whole and is thus checked by negative feedback. To borrow an example from Brody and Sobel, if the heart begins to function irregularly, say by pumping blood too slowly or too rapidly, it will jeopardize the level of blood flow needed by certain organs to perform their functions. This being so, other mechanisms such as neural and hormonal responses are triggered to speed up or to slow down the heart as required, returning the overall system to homeostasis (basic equilibrium). "Positive feedback" refers to the regulation of information flow often associated with growth and maturation. Deviation within the system is thus reinforced and enhanced to promote a change deemed to be beneficial to, or at least not incompatible with, the overall integrity of the integrated whole. The exact nature of information flow will of course vary at each level of organizational complexity. The flow of information at the level of the complex organization of the human species, for example, will almost invariably involve some form of symbolization or linguistic act, whereas the configurations of atoms within molecules will be determined largely by electrostatic attractions and repulsions.

The systems view of life has considerable relevance for the articulation of a philosophical framework within which the concepts of health and disease can be reconceptualized. Consider first that according to the systems view, there is a constant exchange of matter, energy, and information between all living systems and their environments. Given that a living system is self-organizing, its internal order is not imposed by the environment. In this regard, living systems enjoy a certain degree of autonomy, though the exact expression of that autonomy is environmentally influenced. Self-organization does not imply isolation, but it does imply the capacity for self-renewal and self-transcendence. Self-renewal refers to the capacity of the organism within limits to maintain the integrity of its overall organizational pattern despite external stimuli which serve to challenge it. Self-transcendence is rather a vaguer concept, but it implies the capacity on the part of some higher level organisms, as Capra puts it, "to reach out creatively beyond physical and mental boundaries in the processes of learning, development, and evolution." [27]

The counterpart of the notion of self-transcendence in health terms suggests that the interaction between an organism and the environment involves a subtle interplay in which the symbolic value of the interaction for the organism can be sufficiently powerful to transform the resultant effects normally associated with a peculiar environmental stimulus. The "placebo effect," discussed more fully in the Introduction, provides an ample illustration of the point. Placebos are, as we saw, "imitation" or so-called "inactive" medicines, prepared to look authentic so that the patients to whom they are administered believe they are receiving the real thing. The studies considered earlier established that placebos enjoy an impressive degree of success in producing dramatic recoveries from illnesses which - in conventional medical terms - have been pronounced to be curable. By using placebos as a substitute for regular medication in the treatment of a wide range of health problems, we saw that "satisfactory relief" has resulted for 30 percent of the patients taking them. [28]

On the systems view, the concept of health involves far more than the absence of symptoms and signs of disease. [29] Health is construed as a positive and dynamic process in which a living organism, reckoned as an integrated system, is able to respond adaptively to the various environmental states which confront it. [30] These environmental states may range from stress episodes on the one hand to physical, chemical, and even social challenges to the organizational integrity of the system as a whole on the other.

Although the concept of health implies that the system maintains a sense of internal balance, the level of balance associated with health is itself *dynamic* and *changing*, not a static state of equilibrium. Organisms are themselves so interconnected with the environment that they cannot in health terms be separated from it.[31] What happens to the environment is ultimately reflected in some way by the organism, and vice versa.[32] The stability of the system results *not* from its remaining unchanged, but from its capacity to make adaptive changes of such a kind that its total organizational pattern in relation to the environment is preserved despite the fact that its specific components are constantly being replaced.[33] The state of nonequilibrium of a living system is itself a condition of its capacity for self-organization. Without food (i.e., the intake of other ordered structures), for example, living systems would be unable to carry out the internal functions which contribute to their overall organization. In this sense living systems are "open systems" and sustain themselves through a constant exchange of energy and matter with their environment. Chemicals enter and leave the human body at a rate which almost defies credulity. Using radioisotopic techniques, it has been demonstrated, for example, that 98 percent of the 10^{28} atoms which constitute the human body are replaced annually.[34]

Dossey reported that every component within the body exhibits its own patterns of cell renewal and exchange with the elements of the earth, a process he calls the "biodance." Within a week the stomach lining replaces itself; the skin is entirely renewed within a month and the liver is known to regenerate itself within six weeks. Even our genes display an astonishing dynamism. Given that the organic material of which genes are made is protein, the basic component of all genes, DNA, enjoys a relatively short existence of only a few months.[35]

The extent to which the living organism responds adaptively to environmental challenges will determine the resultant level of health experienced by the individual. Adaptive responses may vary in their degree of efficacy. Some adaptations may actually lower the health status of the individual, diminishing the organism's capability of effectively meeting future environmental confrontations, while other adaptations may serve simply to restore the organism to its level of health previous to the challenge, a kind of homeostatic adjustment. The body's healthy response to infection provides a good illustration of the way in which its defenses are engaged through the mobilization of white blood cells which either eradicate the perturbation or at least keep it from spreading.

The concept of disease follows naturally from our discussion. Disease represents the failure of the organism to adapt sufficiently to such perturbation. When this happens, the challenge to the system serves to bring about a disruption of its total pattern of organization. The disruption of the total dynamic balance of the system may result from rigidity in feedback constraints that would otherwise allow for compensatory responses by the component parts. A challenge to the system, in other words, would normally be accommodated by internal adjustments within the system to compensate for the malfunction of one or other of its parts. Disease, however, seems more commonly to result when the perturbation or challenge to the system is so great that even when the normal compensatory and homeostatic mechanisms are functioning properly, the system is unable to produce a sufficiently adaptive response. Although certain perturbation may initially be directed to a particular hierarchical level, the systemic structure of the organism ensures that the disruption will impact - if left unchecked by the appropriate feedback mechanisms - across the entire system. Radiation, for example, impinges initially upon the molecular level, but its prolonged effect is the degradation of every hierarchical level of organization within the system. Having impinged upon the molecular level, disruptions soon occur at the biochemical level which in turn provokes deleterious changes at the cellular level. These aberrations lead to the degeneration of the organ systems whose malfunction contributes to the eventual disruption and dissipation of the overall system of which they are components.

Nor need the chain of systemically correlated events end here. As physiological degeneration occurs, an array of related behavioral modifications and personality changes also occur. The systemic disruption of a disease such as polio, for example, may leave the polio victim disfigured and crippled. Both changes are, as one might imagine, personally devastating and require considerable adaptation to the limitations of freedom and self-expression imposed by the disease. In this regard the twin concepts of health and disease are multifaceted, having both personal and societal aspects. It is *personal* in that the human capacity for work, play, love, and other forms of self-expression are intimately and inextricably bound up with *how* people feel, being conditioned by their actual and their perceived well-being. As physiological, mental, or attitudinal disease transformation occur, the behavioral and personality changes which accompany them in turn impact upon the family, friends and, depending on the circumstances, the community as a whole. Individuals who are severely disabled by disease or illness, for example, are not infrequently dependent upon others, as family members and other social institutions assist with the burden of health care and rehabilitation. Furthermore, some diseases are inherently social by virtue of being perpetuated genetically, as is haemophilia. Inasmuch as other diseases are communicable they can, in a variety of ways, be disruptive of established social harmony. Acquired Immune Deficiency Syndrome offers a current case in point, ranking as a disease having social aspects not only in being communicable but also in being socially provocative and divisive.

Rather than viewing health and disease as diametrically opposed, the two concepts can be seen in a relationship of dynamic interaction such that it may sometimes be difficult to draw a definitive boundary between them.[36] For example, a person may in the traditional sense be suffering from a disease, but given appropriate supports from loved ones, friends, and the community, manifest an attitude which is definitive of the dynamic sense of well-being one would ordinarily associate with those individuals free of disease. Similarly, happiness is not equivalent to health. An individual might, for example, sacrifice health to achieve a goal with which personal happiness is associated. The achievement of a competitive sporting goal such as boxing is a useful example. On the systems view, disease is not to be regarded as *something* a person has, or as a state of incapacitation simply imposed upon a person from outside. As Engel puts it, "disease corresponds to failures or disturbances in growth, development, functions and adjustments of the organism as a whole or any of its systems." [37] On our interpretation of the systems view, the concepts of health and disease are to be regarded as referring to interdependent rather than separate and autonomous states of being. They are different points of reference on the same continuum of systemic configuration.

Prigogine's theory of 'dissipative structures' and the functional interdependence of health and disease

There is another aspect of the interrelation and interdependence between health and disease which marks a radical departure from the conventional bioreductionist construal of these concepts. When the systems interpretation of health and disease is coupled with the work of the late Ilya Prigogine, physicist and winner of the Nobel Prize in 1977, [38] the conceptual offspring produced affords an exciting new view of the constellation of issues which influence our understanding of health and disease. Although it may on first consideration appear to be counterintuitive, the view we now wish to defend affirms that far from being antithetical, health and disease are complicitous in what might be called the process of adaptive evolution. To put it even more strongly, disease and illness are, in an important philosophical sense, preconditions of health. Let us try to relieve the obscurity of this epigram.

Prigogine has been called the "poet of thermodynamics" by the Nobel Committee, and his work has been seen by others as interweaving science and mysticism, and as bridging the traditional hiatus between the biological and social sciences. Of particular relevance for our discussion of health is the purport of his mathematically elegant equations to demonstrate that, according to the systems view, the phenomenon of self organization is not the sole prerogative or monopoly of living organisms but characteristics also certain nonliving systems such as particular chemical reactions.[39] The Zhabotinski chemical reaction is a case in point. [40] In this chemical reaction a systemic process of self-organization occurs in which scroll-like patterns and shapes unfold, while the colors of the solution oscillate, changing from red to blue at regular intervals. Prigogine's research has been concerned primarily to develop a dynamic theory to explicate the logical features of such systems. [41]

He refers to these highly organized but dynamic systems as "dissipative structures," and we will see in what follows that they provide a context of interface with nature previously thought by conventional science to be unavailable. Dissipative structures can thus be seen to provide a nexus of dynamic interrelation between animate and inanimate matter. [42] He writes: "We know we can interact with nature. That is the heart of the message I give. . . Matter is not inert. It is alive and active. Life is always changing one way or another through its adaptation to nonequilibrium conditions."[43]

To understand the force of Prigogine's work and the use which we will make of it respect of the concepts of health and disease, it will be instructive to consider the context in which his ideas take their life. An important feature of the conventional scientific interpretation of the universe is embodied in the Second Law of Thermodynamics, well-known for its pessimistic prediction of the "heat-death" demise of the universe. The basic idea here is that the universe suffers an endemic process of degradation known as "entropy" in which the energy which constitutes the entire universe is "running down" and being irreversibly lost in the form of heat. The final state of this ineradicable heat death is called "equilibrium."

In local defiance of the Second Law of Thermodynamics, the life process seems to be an exception, reflecting through the patterns of evolution presumed to govern its development a trend towards greater complexity. As Dossey remarks, "In a universe that is gradually running downhill, life processes are continually running uphill in defiance of the thermodynamicists' second law."[44] In essence Prigogine's Nobel Prize winning theory is an attempt to reconcile the Second Law of Thermodynamics, and the entropy calculus which derives from it, with the character of biological systems which exhibit a disposition towards greater rather than less complexity. On Prigogine's account entropy does not distribute uniformly across the whole of the universe, but is enfolded in nature in such a way that the instability which it generates is itself the source of energy for the transformation of nature. [45] Fluctuations of energy arising from entropy, that is to say, may result in configurations of energy which constitute new forms of complexity. [46] The important point here is that dissipative structures reorder themselves at higher levels of systemic complexity *because* of entropy, not in spite of it. The life and death processes of the universe are paradoxically part of the same systemic phenomenon. The higher the level of energy transformation, the more - as Prigogine puts it - "life least entropy," not the other way around. The entropic trend towards equilibrium or to the heat death of the entire universe creates the potential for the reorganization at a higher level of complexity of certain parts of it.

According to Prigogine, dissipative structures are *open systems.*[47, 48] Living organisms, even parts of them such as seeds or ova, are examples of open systems. Open systems, or dissipative structures as Prigogine prefers to label them, display the dynamics of self-organization. By breaking down, or utilizing other structures in the environment as a source of energy, dissipative structures maintain or transform themselves, discarding or returning to the environment the degraded waste which results from the process of dissipative metabolism taking place within them. [49] Prigogine provides the example of a town as a highly complex dissipative structure which utilizes energy from the surrounding environs (e.g., raw materials, fossil fuels, etc.), transforms it into a new complex structure, say an industrial complex, and returns energy to the environment in the form of waste.

Unlike a closed system, of which a rock could be an example, open systems are engaged in a continuous exchange of energy with the environment. The more complex the structure, the more energy is required to preserve its coherence, in part because, this being so, there are more interrelations to sustain the further it is from equilibrium. The further from equilibrium a system is the more vulnerable it is to internal fluctuations, and depending upon the extent of the perturbation to the system, its structural integrity is maintained or altered. Because the degree of complexity determines the degree of systemic vulnerability, each energy transformation makes the next one likelier. Hence, the greater the proclivity to entropic disorganization, or as it may otherwise be put, the greater the proclivity to disentropic reorganization. Order and chaos are not, as the conventional wisdom would have us believe, diametrically opposed; they are rather cooperative aspects within the same continuum of process, much as we described the concepts of health and disease earlier.

In sum, the heuristic paradox which arises out of Prigogine's theory affirms that the more complex, intricately interconnected, and coherent a dissipative structure is, the more dependent it becomes upon an increasing flow of energy from the environment to sustain it. The higher the degree of complexity, the more likely it becomes that internal perturbations can act as catalysts to reformation or higher-level adaptation within the system. Ferguson puts the point well:

> At first the idea of creating new order by perturbation seems outrageous, like shaking up a box of random words and pouring out a sentence. Yet our traditional wisdom contains parallel ideas. We know that stress often forces sudden new solutions; that crisis often alerts us to opportunity; that the creative

process requires chaos before form emerges; that individuals are often strengthened by suffering and conflict; and that societies need a healthy airing of dissent . . . .

We are transformed through interaction with the environment. Science can now express as beautifully as the humanities the great and final paradox: our need to connect with the world (relationship) and to define our unique position in it (autonomy). [50]

The initial relevance of Prigogine's theory to the area of health should now be obvious. Extending the theory of dissipative structures, it is clear that encounters with environmental challenges, including disease, may prompt a creative adaptation within the living system which leaves the system stronger than it was previously. Exposure to certain disease perturbations - while for a time causing disorder and chaos - can actually serve to raise the health status of the particular organism to a new and higher level of function, say in its immunity to disease. We are unwittingly transformed to a greater or lesser degree through our interaction with the environment, and the dynamic state of health which results from this interchange incorporates the challenge of disease perturbation as a condition of its function. The notion of a disease-free existence is, on the systems view of health we are defending, a contradiction in terms. A certain level of disease perturbation is itself the catalyst to the transformation achieved in obtaining a higher level of health.

Not all perturbations of course are beneficial to the functional well-being of the living organism. Some threats to health are more than the body can bear and in such cases disease perturbation may involve the fundamental disruption of the overall pattern of systemic organization, thereby causing death. Immunization is a process which trades upon the interface between health and disease, between stability and vulnerability. Immunization entails the artificial or deliberate introduction of altered micro-organisms or "disease entities" into the body, the result of which is to challenge the body to respond adaptively by producing antibodies to protect us against the particular disease should we encounter it in the future. Too minor a perturbation will allow the system's feedback mechanism to stifle the effects of the innoculum, thereby pre-empting the immune system response with its entourage of relevant antibodies. On the other hand, too great a perturbation can - far from stimulating an adaptive resistance pattern to the disease - actually stimulate the disease itself. The interface between health and disease which contributes to the increased adaptive complexity of the organism is thus a delicate equilibrium to be respected and preserved. Well-being is the result of the complementary systemic interactions of adaptation and perturbation.[51] In the paradoxical sense of Prigogine's dissipative structures, health and disease constitute a functional process of complementarity. Dossey remarks in this connection:

If we were never perturbed by illness, could we *ever* be healthy? If we never knew illness we would likely lack a corresponding notion of health. . . .There is reason to believe that our body *feeds* on illness to create health, just as dissipative structures "eat entropy," or disorganization, as Schrödinger

> maintained, in this evolution toward increasing complexity. . . .Health is impossible without disturbances, although we traditionally think it is impossible with disturbances. [52]

The systems approach to health care

On the systems view the bioreductionist model focuses upon the lower levels of the organizational hierarchy of living systems, namely physiochemical dysfunction. In the light of the foregoing discussion of the multifaceted character of disease perturbation, it should be clear that even ailments presented primarily as somatic complaints exhibit patterns of disruption which impact across the entire system. If medical intervention is appropriate, it will be directed to different levels of systemic organization assimilated into a program of *total* patient care afforded, as we will see in later chapters, by some primary health care systems. It may be that a therapy aimed at one level of organizational integrity will have therapeutic repercussions across the system. As Brody and Sobel write:

> The systems view also avoids the problem of confusing the level of intervention with the level of disease. While diseases may represent patterns of disruption affecting many hierarchical levels, a therapy aimed at one level may be highly efficacious because it can affect other levels via the interconnected patterns of information flow. Thus, chemotherapy for depression is often strikingly effective even though depressive disorders are characterized by complex mixtures of genetic, biochemical, behavioral, and social factors. Therefore, to conclude from a clinical trial of a drug that depression is only a biochemical disease would be to ignore the true complexity of the illness. [53]

In the light of Prigogine's illumination of certain aspects of systems theory in relation to dissipative structures, it is evident that the goal of health cannot - as the conventional wisdom supposes - be equivalent to the total eradication of disease and illness. The deeper question posed by his work is the extent to which educating for health can facilitate the dynamic of adaptation to disease and illness perturbation. This involves a radically different posture towards health. For the most part conventional health care is designed to help the patient battle against illness, using the ever-growing arsenal of drugs, diagnostic procedures, and tests, injections, and surgery. The quest for health has traditionally been regarded as the battle *against* disease. We struggle, that is to say, to avoid disease and to eschew disruption of any kind to the organizational integrity of the living organism. In the struggle to be free of disease we lose sight of the fact that our defense mechanisms against disease have evolved through encounters of disease perturbation. There is no world free of disease, for without the mechanisms of the auto-immune system, the environment would as a whole be disease-threatening. It is precisely our successfully adaptive encounters with perturbation which have saved us from the nightmare of immune deficiency in a world of multifarious pathogens. As Dossey suggests:

> Our health strategy needs to incorporate flexibility as a primary goal - the adaptability and capacity to react to the periodic challenges to our body-mind integrity. What we do in the interval *between* illness also becomes crucial. I can, by conscious effort, sabotage my body's wisdom to resist perturbations. If I subject myself to negative habits - smoking, obesity, unrelieved exposure to stress, chronic fatigue, failure to exercise, uninterrupted anxiety or depression - I limit my body's homeostatic capacity to react to external perturbations. . . Seen from this perspective, the *real* medicine is what we do *between* illness-events. [54]

Although there are some perturbations so catastrophic that they require direct intervention to deal with them, it is clear that most of what constitutes illness and disease is not of this kind. We have the power to shape our health by becoming wiser about the things that make us unhealthy, but we need also to augment the body's wisdom by cultivating the dynamics of adaptive efficacy to perturbations which cannot by avoided.

The twenty first century is plagued with perturbations which characterize different aspects of our contemporary lifestyle and of life itself. Crowded cities, competition at virtually every level of human interchange, unemployment, war, personal conflicts, and the suffering and deaths of loved ones are just a few of the experiences capable of producing stress. The *specific* responses to environment "stressors" may of course vary considerably. Not all *potential* perturbations are *actual* perturbations, internalized as negative factors in personal health. How disruptive an experience is will depend upon the nature of the experience, including its duration, the individual's perception of the experience, and the capacity to control and shape positive responses to events. Inasmuch as a perturbation could force a degree of reorganization within the system which in turn serves to enhance the overall functioning of the system, stress could actually benefit the organism by increasing its level of complexity.

High-tech culture and the stress factor in disease

There is a subtle ambiguity in the use of the term "stress." It refers on the one hand to individual *responses* in the form of manifested mental states such as "anxiety" and "fear" to any of a range of environmental stimuli such as traffic congestion, loud noises and, more profoundly, the death of a loved one. In this sense stress is a fundamentally *subjective* phenomenon. Two individuals, for example, might both be victims of the same train crash, yet respond to the trauma of the event in entirely different ways. Being trapped in a wrecked carriage might for one individual prove to be ineradicably stressful, while for the other individual, the experience could be perceived as an adventure - exciting but not stressful in the negative mode. If an individual were contemplating suicide, the crash might even by welcomed. How one *perceives* the events of one's life will thus make a great difference as to how one *experiences* them. The emphasis here is on the meaning we attach and the value we give to the environmental stimuli awaiting our response.

On the other hand there are certain events which by their very nature would on any account seem somehow to be *objectively* stressful. The emphasis here is on the events themselves rather than on the individual's perception of them. This is not to say that the way in which the individual perceives the event will not make a difference as to the experience of it. It is to say that some environmental stimuli are stressful independently of our interpreting them as such. While we may not regard the presence of chemicals such as chlorine in our water as a source of worry and stress, such chemicals place a physiological stress on the central nervous system which impacts in turn throughout the various subsystems of the entire organism. Stress is significant in understanding disease processes when we appreciate that stress is a *psychosocial* factor which makes the greatest sense in the context of the psychological and sociological factors which influence the physiological processes of disease.[55]

In 1936 Hans Selye initiated an investigation into the effect of different forms of stress on living organisms. It has been reported that his initial investigations prompted a series of studies which have led to some 150,000 publications.[56, 57] One of the earliest connections to be established between stress and disease concerned the suppression of the immune system as a consequence of undergoing the trauma of bereavements. It was Dr. C. Murray Parkes, a British physician who in collaboration with a research team from the Tavistock Institute of Human Relations in London published a persuasive study of 4,448 widowers of fifty-five years or older, monitoring their health for a period of nine years subsequent to the death of the spouse. The startling conclusion of the study stated that widowers were five times more likely to die within six months of the deaths of their wives than would otherwise be the case.[58]

Equally interesting is the fact that the majority of widowers who died within the six-month period died of the *same* disease which killed their wives. There are many hypotheses advanced to explain these correlations, including the view that during the grief period widowers are far more likely to drink and smoke heavily, rely more on pills and tranquilizers than usual, exercise less, socialize less, sleep less, and even eat less. There is also evidence to show that as the impact of the aftershock of grief diminishes, the level of immune system integrity returns to pre-bereavement levels. This data is encouraging, for it reveals a delicate equilibrium between stress and immune system function such that by reducing the stress responsible for suppression of the immune system, it is possible to restore the system to its original state. Steven Locke and Douglas Colligan of the Harvard Medical School have shown that, in the face of stress, "good copers" displayed significantly higher immune function than did "poor copers."[59, 60] Inasmuch as they have also demonstrated that we can to some extent learn to manage stress situations, the function of the immune system is not entirely outside our control. The traditional view has been that the immune system functioned, not unlike the kidneys or liver, as an involuntary or self-regulating system. Pioneering work on stress management proves that we are far more in control of our own health - even the subtle workings of the immune system - than the conventional wisdom has supposed. The role of altered awareness as a factor in the processes of health and disease could well by regarded as a fundamental tenet of the wholistic health movement.

Terms and expressions have been coined to heighten consciousness of the extent to which, though we cannot avoid certain "stressors" in our lives, we can control or at least minimize their negative impact upon us. The recognition of the degree of control we have in respect of stress management is implied by expressions such as "restful alertness," "passive volition," "deliberate letting," "giving-in," and "acquiescence." The possibility of managing stress is part and parcel of paying attention to it. Or to put it differently, the *refusal* to confront stress is itself a *form of stress.* Becoming more aware of the stressors confronting us, doing what we can to remove and control them is crucial to the maintenance of health and the prevention of disease. The body and mind act as one united front in the management of health. Our responses to stress and the analysis of these responses show that in subtle ways we have the power of mind to make ourselves well or to let ourselves succumb to sickness. As Ferguson insightfully writes:

> The old saying, "name your poison," applies to the semantics and symbols of disease. If we feel "picked on" or someone gives us a pain in the neck, we may make our metaphors literal—with acne or neck spasms. People have long spoken of a "broken heart" as the result of a disappointing relationship; now research has shown a connection between loneliness and heart disease. In animal research, heart disease has been caused by the prolonged stimulation of a brain region associated with strong emotion. The same region is connected to the immune system. So the "broken heart" may become coronary disease; the need to grow may become a tumor, the ambivalence a "splitting headache," the rigid personality arthritis. Every metaphor is potentially a literal reality. [61]

The actual physiological mechanism by way of which stress impacts on our well-being are not entirely clear, but there is considerable evidence drawn from animal studies to show that on the surfaces of lymphocytes - the central immune system cells - are receptors to which hormones and neuro-transmitter chemicals from the brain attach to influence the function of the immune system. When a person is under certain kinds of stress, the cerebral cortex (the conscious brain) is thought to stimulate the hypothalamus, which in turn activates and regulates the hormones and neurotransmitters responsible for immune system efficacy. The impact on the immune system of acute versus chronic stress is less clear, but it is incontestable that stressors such as bereavement are associated with the increased incidence of disease and increased mortality. It is, as we observed earlier, established also that bereavement is associated with the suppression of the immune system. What remains to be demonstrated is the exact link between the lowered immune system function of the widowers and the specific diseases which caused their deaths.

That stress management is a key factor in the maintenance of health and the prevention of disease, however, is unequivocal, as are certain of the psychosocial patterns which are inherently stressful and in respect of which we organize our lives. A considerable literature has accumulated, for example, to show that some of the most common causes of death in our society such as atherosclerotic heart disease and cancer are associated with particular personality types, [62] classified as more or less stressed by their own perceptions of psychosocial factors as seemingly innocuous as time. Within contemporary society we have in large part structured our lives by the clock. We have in effect become slaves to time, though time is in essence a construct of our own invention. We get up by the clock, usually start and finish work by the clock, choose our entertainment by the clock, and generally rush to live our lives by the clock. The constraints on our lives imposed by time represent not just a specific aspect of stress but rather a whole framework of organizational patterns within which sundry aspects of stress derive their negative force. Elucidation of this point may be instructive.

It is to be admitted at the outset that there are different logical categories of time-experience. Nevertheless, it is clear that the commonsense view of time expresses time- experience in terms of past, present, and future events. Once the impetus to reductionism takes over in the analysis of time, we see these conventional divisions giving way to the finer descriptions of their constituents and we find ourselves talking about temporal structures such as millennia, centuries, decades, years, months, weeks, days, hours, moments, seconds, and so on. The conventional disposition has been to divide time into finer and finer slices. Whether we view time according to this disposition as linear or cyclic depends upon the devices used to designate periodicity. [63]

For many ancient and indeed some primitive cultures today, time is demarcated by successions in nature such as the varying but repeating phases of the moon or the periodic flooding of rivers. Discriminations by appeal to successions in nature fostered the idea of time as a cyclic phenomenon, and devices such as the sundial were invented with circular scales to measure it. As our ancestors felt more in control of nature, however, one can imagine that they began to feel less compelled to rely on its characteristics to define their relationship to it. Inasmuch as technology gave power *over* nature, it was to technology that they turned to define the categories by virtue of which to understand it. Devices for measuring the periodicity of time thus came to reflect the current state of technological control over nature. By way of the *technology* of time-telling, for example, we have as a society now abandoned our reliance upon nature's periodicities in favor of the periodicities of our own artifacts, e.g., from the time it takes a candle to burn to the atomic interactions of a cesium clock. The shift of categorical interpretation and representation from the cycles of nature to man-made measures of periodicity encouraged a radical reconception of the logical character of time. The concept of time as cyclic gave way to its redefinition as a flowing, asymmetric, and linear phenomenon not to be repeated. [64]

With these changes in our concept of time came changes in our relationship to nature. The more we become dominated by the technology of chronometrics, for instance, the less attuned we become not only to the cycles in nature but to the cycles and biorhythms in ourselves. For the most part we no longer eat when we are hungry or sleep when we are sleepy, but eat and sleep according to the technological devices we have invented to measure time. We become dominated not by time *per se*, but by our concept of it; not as time manifests itself in the patterns of nature but as manifested in the patterns of our technology which reflect the way in which we see nature. The technology we have used to dominate nature has thus come paradoxically to dominate us and our categories of self-understanding. In this sense the "watch" is well-named; in that we use it to watch our lives pass according to the time *it keeps*. On Gottlieb's view the watch is in essence a symbol of death. Wedged in between birth and death, we coordinate our lives to the relentless flow of our watches and clocks. We literally *watch* our lives passing by, for we have unwittingly committed ourselves to a linear and reductionist view of nature in which time is running out and will never return. [65] At a fundamental level of the unconscious we have structured our experience of nature in spatiotemporal terms which ensure that we are constantly witnessing our own deaths. In a bizarre way we have transformed life itself into the medium for the experience of our own deaths. With every tick of the clock we are covertly reminded of our finitude and mortality; we *watch* our youth escaping us with every passing moment, and every passing second is a second closer to death. When we think of our health on this model of time, we are led ineluctably to associate our health with the passing of our youth. Reductionist time flow betrays our commitment to entropy; not only are our lives "running down," but so is the whole of reality. We are strangely caught in a Catch-22 of our own making: the more we attend to our health, the more aware we become of its inevitable and real decline and our ever-increasing proximity to death.

The presumption that time is linear and infinitely divisible underpins our basic conceptions of life and death and of health and disease. It is the central contention of this section that our *perception* of the reality of time as entropic is such a fundamental conceptual feature of the principles by way of which we organize the world that we literally mirror this perception in the function of our internal organs and bodily processes and thus in the state of our health. Believing that time is running out, that we are pitted against the entropic clock of nature, we generate - unwittingly or wittingly - maladies in our own bodies which are validations of this belief. We become what Friedman and Rosenman call "time-sick" or Type A individuals who orient their lives around goals, deadlines, and hard and fast objectives. [66] They live their lives according to the clock and the calendar. They are consumed *not* so much by the love of their work, which is timeless, but by their sense of temporal urgency, which is not. They are disposed to doing everything rapidly; they work, eat, and even sleep hurriedly. Type A individuals are on the whole ambitious and highly successful; they are what Friedman and Rosenman call "striving personalities." Although they are generally admired for their accomplishments, they exhibit as a group a characteristic that is unenviable - they are possessed of a higher mortality rate from coronary heart disease than those groups which do not display the same sense of inner urgency. As a group, they exhibit significantly high elevations in heart rate and blood pressure, adrenalin, insulin, hydrocortisone, along with significantly increased respiratory rates, secretions of gastric acid, secretory activity, blood cholesterol, and muscle tension. According to Friedman and Rosenman, over 90 percent of the males less than sixty years of age who have heart attacks display "Type A" behavior, a clear indictment of the negative impact of stress factors associated with the linear conception of time. [67, 68]

But do we need to accept the reductionist conception of time as linear and entropic? This is a question we will answer in the negative, and we begin our reply by making explicit an aspect of Prigogine's work which thus far has only been implicit. In his description of the transformation of dissipative structures Prigogine avers that his equations presuppose that the whole process of systemic patterns of organization is *nonlinear.* He compares dissipative structural processes to driving in heavy freeway traffic. When the traffic is light, one is at liberty to drive in a linear way, being obliged to slow and to change lanes only occasionally. Once the traffic becomes heavy, one is no longer simply driving; one is in an important sense being driven by the system of traffic of which one is a part. All the cars are affecting each other; to speak of singular, linear movement is to simplify the systemic interactions to the point of distortion. [69] The point can be extended to advance our understanding of time stressors.

If our perception of time is reconceptualized in such a way that time is not a linear "quantity" which is constantly running out, then we may find ourselves running less and *stressing ourselves less* to catch up with it. The capacity to relax is tantamount to "slowing time" partly by reconceptualizing it and partly by reconceptualizing our relation to it. This may be one reason why relaxation techniques such as meditation have proved so successful in reducing stress and the range of medical conditions associated with it. The work of Herbert Benson of the Harvard Medical School has been pioneering in this connection. His books on the "relaxation response" are particularly useful in understanding the impressive contribution which can be made to health by relaxation techniques. [70] In a study carried out by Wallace and Benson, Transcendental Meditation (TM) proved capable of reducing the subjects' respiratory rates, along with heart rates, cardiac output, oxygen consumption, and carbon dioxide elimination. The simultaneous rise in skin resistance confirmed that these changes were accompanied by a reduction of stress. It was also found that in a survey of 394 meditators, 67 percent reported improvements in their physical health, and 84 percent reported improvements in their mental well-being. Other studies have shown that meditators report a larger decrease of usage than nonmeditators of addictive drugs, ranging from alcohol and marijuana to LSD and heroin, a decrease in the usage of hypertensive medication, and a reduction in reports of somatic symptoms. [71, 72]

Meditation has been shown to be a beneficial strategy for the management of a number of clinical and health-related problems. Its efficacy in comparison to other self-regulating strategies for stress management is encouraging, but more research needs to be done in this area to clarify ambiguities in the analysis of its clinical effectiveness. That meditation works to reduce stress by enhancing the relaxed state indicates that the reconceptualization and reorganization of our patterns of lifestyle which make us tense and unrelaxed must also be addressed. The potentially oppressive restrictions of the clock can undermine our health as assuredly as can trauma of life. Ultimately, health will depend upon the capacity of an organism to adapt constructively to environmental stressors on the one hand, and upon the capacity of the community and society to ensure that the stressors which we cannot avoid and which are of our own making do not dissipate the human organism beyond the point of its potential for compensatory restoration and growth on the other.

Summary

In the present chapter we have considered the traditional definitions of health and disease and have found them deficient on several counts. We observed that inasmuch as modern medical science adheres to a limited view of biology which is quantitative and reductionistically oriented, the concept of health as the absence of disease unsurprisingly reflects the impoverished philosophy of medical scientism which underpins it. The growing commitment to wholistic health signals a salutary corrective to the myopia of modern medical scientism.

In the light of the philosophical framework of the previous chapter we considered the relevance of the systems view of life as providing an alternative and wholistic perspective on health. We saw that on the systems view, self-organizing systems are characterized by hierarchical levels and a fundamental interdependency among them. Rather than being regarded as a monolithic relation between signs and symptoms on the one hand and micro-organisms on the other, disease is construed on the systems model as a failure of adaption to an environmental challenge which in consequence causes disruption to the integrity of the living system. Patterns of disruption cannot be confined to a particular level of organizational complexity, as what impinges on one level in turn impacts upon the others. Ultimately, health is a global matter.

We considered also the work of the Nobel prizewinner, Ilya Prigogine, whose work has shown that dissipative structures are open systems engaged in constant interchange with the environment. Always in process, the system is constantly changing, with certain fluctuations of energy resulting in perturbations to the integrity of the system as a whole. Depending upon the level of perturbation and its intensity, the living system may reorder itself in such a way as to achieve a higher level of complexity and adaptability to environmental challenge. We also observed the relevance of Prigogine's theory to the philosophy of health and to the wholistic approach to health care. It was argued that health and disease are not diametrically opposed but can be seen as complementary components in a total process of organizational development.

Finally, we considered the psychosocial phenomenon of stress as a significant factor in ill health and disease. We saw that stress awareness is the first step in stress management, and we considered the example of "time-sickness" as a part of the hidden agenda of the framework within which as a society we organize our lifestyle in healthy and unhealthy ways. Finally, we looked briefly at meditation as a self-regulating strategy for the management of stress, showing that its success depends partly upon the recognition that we are, as a culture, "time-sick." Meditation proves to provide a way of coping with stress, but it was also observed that the management of stress must extend to the eradication of its causes. We will in the next chapter examine more closely some of those causes.

CHAPTER 4

The theory of transformative subjugation and understanding its ramifications for integrated well-being

Our previous explorations of the foundations of wholistic medicine, and of the concepts of health and disease which follow from them, confirm that the advancement of community health depends primarily upon a profoundly ecological understanding of the conditions under which the goal of health for all can be achieved. The medium for the promotion of health is neither improved medical technology nor the ever-increasing magic of the doctor's scalpel - it is education. Our major task as a society is to provide the educational context and resources by way of which the physical, biological, and social forces which impact upon health can be understood and managed through adaptation and reform. We have seen that "health" is not so much a *state* of well-being as a *process* of well-being, a potentiality in respect of which individuals and the community adapt to their surroundings to maximize the full range of biological and psychosocial functions which define them as human.

As a species, we are capable of acquiring or developing a remarkable tolerance towards environmental conditions as diverse as pollution, contamination of food and water, lack of physical activity, etc. Nonetheless, there are limits to the adaptations we can make to the world in which we find ourselves and to which a large part is of our own making. Certain mechanisms of human adaptation are simply circumscribed by our genetic program. We are genetically programmed, that is to say, to tolerate only so much radiation or chemical contamination; beyond the threshold of adaptation, the compensatory function of the organism is defunct. Sociocultural forces may in sundry ways serve also to distort the adaptive mechanisms which do exist. The multiple stress factors which pervade our big cities, for example, have a *cumulative* effect which may serve to undermine the organism's capacity to respond adaptively to any one such stressor on its own. The organism's defenses are simply overwhelmed by being outnumbered. Similarly, the accelerated pace of technological change makes it extremely difficult and sometimes impossible for human beings geared biologically to a slower pace of adaptive response, to tolerate the panoply of new substances and environmental modifications never encountered in their biological past. The water we drink, the food we eat, the lifestyle we live have all changed in ways which require our immediate recognition and response if we are to parry their negative influence on health. In this present chapter we shall introduce the concept of "transformative subjugation" and show its relevance for understanding the problem of environmental health risks.

The theory of transformative subjugation

According to what might be termed 'the dominant paradigm of educational epistemology' the objectivity of scientific knowledge ensures that what we know is value-free, as is the technology which derives from it. The idea here is that what we come to know is neither good nor bad, but rather value-neutral.[1] It is how people use knowledge and the technological innovations to which it gives rise that determines its moral status. This point is popularly put euphemistically when it is said, 'Guns don't kill people; people kill people with guns'. While we have no wish to deny that there is a truth in this way of looking at the matter, we shall in what follows be concerned to establish that there is a much deeper and more comprehensive truth which it conceals. The implications of this deeper truth have monumental implications for understanding the covert values which are structurally enshrined in our system of education and our understanding of health.

Part of the problem is that so much of research is spent addressing the issues surrounding how we can effectively transmit knowledge that far too little research is undertaken on what knowledge is and especially, on its impact on the subtler aspects of how we relate to the world around us and to each other. On the conventional presumption that knowledge is in any case value-free there is obviously little sense of personal responsibility on the part either of those who 'discover' it, or of those who teach it, to worry about whether what they discover or teach as knowledge is truly worth discovering or teaching at all. Having failed to make these distinctions explicit and then to explore them philosophically, we have, as a society, become woefully ignorant of the foundational values which have covertly come to define the context for education.

It is tempting to think that scientific knowledge is somehow outside the bounds of intellectual history in the sense of having avoided the 'contamination' of such influences as socio-cultural prejudices, religious assumptions, mythology, and politics, to name only a few. Reflection upon the development of contemporary empiricist science, however, makes palpably clear that all pretence of its virgin birth is misleading and meretricious, as has been pointed out in both chapters 1 and 2. Despite its pretensions to methodological purity and the virginal symbolism of the 'white coats' worn by scientists who inadvertently parade it, the ascension of the highly quantified formulation of knowledge proffered in our educational institutions is not without its own historical biography of conceptual dogmatism, religious fanaticism, gender bias, and vested interests.

Similarly, the political history which reflects the attempts of science to discredit and systematically eliminate a number of unorthodox aspirants to the crown of knowledge itself constitutes an important facet of the historical development of the dominant paradigm of science. Despite its privileged position of epistemic priority, the dominant paradigm of knowledge may arguably be more socio-culturally entrenched than epistemically entrenched. In the West scientific knowledge in its empiricist, quantitative and statistical guise has been socially legitimated as the ultimate standard against which other aspirants to the accolade of knowledge are to be measured. However, the dominant paradigm of knowledge is arguably as much a cultural phenomenon as it is a philosophically justified conceptual scheme. In this sense the logical priority we ascribe to it is at least partly gratuitous and needs to be recognized. Doing so makes a significant difference not only to how we come to know the world, but to what it is we come to know.

Far from being 'neutral', every piece of information which is accepted as knowledge is what we shall call here 'structurally encoded' to ensure a covert measure of control over every aspect of our lives. And if the primary form of knowledge we transmit is conditioned and shaped by our obsession with power, both its form and application will reflect the value we place on power and dominance. If what we claim to know, that is to say, is defined implicitly by the capacity of what is 'known' to provide us a power advantage over the world in which we live, the orthodox educational view that knowledge is neither good nor bad in itself can be exposed for the illusion it is.

In the light of the ideological dimensions of the presumption of knowledge encoded as power, we shall argue that there exists within the educational curriculum a conceptually endogenous bias in favor of an epistemology, not only of domination, but of subjugation, and that subjugation is itself a value term which has monumental ramifications for the way in which education actually informs and shapes the very foundations of socio-cultural values.

When knowledge is itself substantively defined by the preoccupation with power, dominance and control, the resultant form of knowledge will enshrine as a fundamental educational value the propriety of subjugation as the measure of our interaction with the world around us and each other.

> "The scientific method...reflects our consuming passion for predictability and order. We have transformed all of physical reality into a giant testing site and then attempted to discover predictable patterns of behavior that can be exploited over and over in such a way as to advance our control over the forces of nature. The more successful we are at imperializing our environment, the more secure we feel".[2]

From this it follows that independently of the 'good intentions' of the persons who utilize the technologies which derive from a theory of knowledge driven by a lust for power, virtually every application of that form of knowledge will in some covert way serve the aim of 'knowing', only insofar as it guarantees a measure of dominance, control and subjugation.

As Laura and Marchant contend;

> "by obliging schoolchildren around the globe to think primarily and increasingly in ways that are circumscribed by the machines we create, we have also covertly encouraged in our schools an invidious conformity of *thinking* about the world in *machine-like* ways. By virtue of the process of reinforcing a

> progressive movement towards the intellectual conformity which results from seeing the world through the 'eyes' of the computer, education has coincidentally encouraged progressive movement towards the demise of intellectual imagination. If there is a difference between indoctrination and education, it must surely lie in the different things we do either to stimulate and nurture the intellectual imagination or to stifle and diminish it".[3]

What we have as a culture failed largely to acknowledge is that the price we pay for this measure of control is the ecological desacrilization of nature, the depersonalization and increasing dehumanization of our relationships, coupled with bizarre modalities of socio-cultural alienation. This is an enormously complex insight, and we make no pretence that in the space available to us here that we shall be able adequately to develop the argument which sustains it. It is to be hoped, none the less, that the fragments of insight we are able to weave with tolerable conceptual coherence will serve to prompt debate and accordingly, future opportunity for us and others to elucidate more satisfactorily these important issues.

According to R. S. Laura, the process of "transformative subjugation" is the logical outcome of embracing a form of knowledge motivated by our insatiable appetite for power. In essence we socially legitimate our craving for power by enshrining it in a way of knowing the world designed to control and dominate it. While he admits that there are many plausible explanations for this preoccupation with power, one of the most alluring is the idea that the more we can dominate and control the natural, socio-cultural , political and economic environment in which we find ourselves, the more secure we can make ourselves feel.

On Laura's view we do this by making the world around us as predictable as possible. The more predictable a thing, process or event is the more control we have over it and thus the more secure we think we become. What follows from this recognition becomes particularly interesting for those of us concerned to explore the reciprocal nexus between education and the epistemological value presumptions to which it gives rise. From this perspective we submit that educational epistemology can be construed as tantamount to an ideological posture.

Because the pragmatic goal of this educational epistemology is to make the world as predictable as possible, the world is essentially stripped of its qualitative dimensions so that what remains for analysis are the quantitative components amenable to calculable precision or in some cases precise probability. The more quantitative a domain, the more readily can its subject matter be subsumed under the laws of science. The more amenable a subject-matter is to scientific laws which ensure predictability, the more objective, or so the power-based scientific epistemology would contend, are the empirical investigations undertaken. What is not amenable to quantification is relegated to the subjective domain of thought, however interesting its ratiocinations might be. To put another gloss on this point, the subject-matter of science reduces to a universe of discourse in which every claim to knowledge is 'entitled' by virtue of being quantifiable. What falls outside the aegis of quantifiable science becomes the subjective prerogative of the arts, metaphysics or sheer nonsense. Given what is now fashionably termed as 'accountability', is it any surprise to be faced increasingly with such conspicuous disparities in funding for these respective enterprises, especially within universities? Although this is admittedly an argument for another occasion, it should none the less be useful to make explicit the present epistemological considerations which prompt the distinction between the arts and science in the first place.

Let us now revert to our discussion of the other value-considerations associated with the dominant theory of knowledge and the theory of transformative subjugation. Given that the primary form of knowledge which underpins the curriculum is driven by our obsession as a culture with power and dominance, much of the technology which follows from it will be designed and deployed in ways that allow us to restructure the world so that it suits our interests. This being so, our interactions with nature and the cultural determinants of the value we place upon it, are subsumed under our technological attempts to reconstruct the world to make it oblige more readily to submit to our will. This process means, so it would seem, that we can spend less of our time having to adapt to the world around us, while spending more of our time enjoying the world we have fabricated to adapt to us. When night falls upon us sooner than we would like, we deploy our technologies of power to turn night into day by artificially lighting our world. If our homes, workplaces or means of transport are hotter or colder than we would like, we create technologies to turn warmth into cold or cold into warmth. When our food crops do not grow fast enough, or as abundantly as we would like, we coax them into obedience by chemically fertilizing the soil in which they grow, or by genetically engineering the plants themselves to grow faster, get bigger and to produce more to eat. If the food we harvest does not transport well, we simply engineer it to make it travel better and still look great; so the tomatoes thus conformed have skins not unlike durable plastic, are big, red and beautiful, but have lost that beautiful tomato flavor and fragrance that make them worth eating in the first place. If our foods do not have a shelf-life long enough to maximize the financial return they bring, we either irradiate them with nuclear energy, dose them with preservatives to inhibit their demise, or cover them in ways to maintain the appearance of a freshness which in fact they no longer have. For other foods such as bread we technologize them by removing from them the very parts (and nutrient components) which define them as alive. Thus, in the technologization of bread, the wheat germ or living kernel of wheat is excised to ensure that a once living loaf of bread is converted into a fabricated product so processed and inert that it has become almost invulnerable to decay. All of which have a detrimental effect on our health.

According to the theory of transformative subjugation, the way in which technology achieves this measure of control is not only to transform the living things of nature into things which are synthesized, artificial and inert, but further to take the things we have fabricated and convert them into other things which are ever more processed, chemicalized and inert. Within the context of the epistemology of power, the covert preoccupation with dominance and control – a fundamental value presupposition in itself – is attained by means of technological transformations which reconstruct the living world in such a way that the behavior of the fabricated things produced can be subsumed under laws of nature. For the more alive and vital a system is, the more difficult it is to predict and control its behaviors. On the other hand, the more inert our technology can make the world and the more synthetic and chemicalized are its components, the easier it is to manipulate the components in ways that make their relationships to each other sufficiently determinate to predict and thus control their behaviors. The paradox or antinomy of the epistemology of power process is that our technologies of power succeed in providing us a measure of predictable control of the world around us only by transforming the world into a fabricated museum of quantitatively regimented, chemicalized, increasingly inert and all too often dead things. The paradox is that the technological kingdom of which we have become rulers is not the living world per se, but the fabricated world of chemicalized, inert and lifeless things of our own making.

Having welcomingly surrounded ourselves with so many of our lifeless fabrications, is it any wonder that we should feel increasingly less healthy, less vital, less connected and less spiritually alive than ever.

The problem with our unwitting commitment to this epistemology of power and the transformative subjugations of technologies which derive from it is not just the obvious ramifications which relate to our systematic desacrilization of nature. Neither is the problem simply the resultant despoiling of our lakes and rivers, our toxic assault upon our seas, the pollution of the air we breathe and the water we drink, the mindless rape of the earth's forests, land and soil, as horrendous and egregious a wounding of the earth that these violations represent. The ramifications of transformative subjugation are far more pernicious and relate to the philosophy of value which the technology of transformative subjugation presupposes. The particular theory of knowledge we have institutionally entrenched within our educational system is far from an innocent and innocuous way of knowing the world.

The epistemology of power enshrined within it is a fundamental presumption of the value of power and dominance, and the underpinning of an ideological posture which aggrandizes gratuitously the freedom human kind has to desacrilze and denigrate the earth as a resource for its own ends. Along with society's commitment to the technologization of nature is the value system which the process of transformative subjugation entails. The values of power, dominance, expropriation of environmental and human resources, if not the presumed right to play God, are deeply embedded within the curriculum, not necessarily explicitly, but covertly as a feature of the hidden agenda which defines the more general goals of education itself.

> "If there is a critical urgency confronting educators, it is to redefine our relationship to nature and to each other by redefining the fundamental concept of educational knowledge in a way which dignifies rather than diminishes our humanity by doing so".[4]

If our technological interventions are implicitly designed to deconstruct the 'living world' so that its components can be used to fabricate a far more synthesized, chemicalized and inert world of predictable outcome, then the hidden agenda of education is on this occasion, in desperate need of critical reflection and assessment. Let us now consider the magnitude of the environmental crisis as it pertains to health with the aim of making this argument clear.

Basic human needs

Maslow believed that a prerequisite for individual development was the satisfaction of the more basic human needs, commencing with the requirements for survival, including water, food, and adequate shelter. Such needs are also those which must be met if an individual is to be born healthy and to maintain his/her health throughout life.

Nutrition

Without adequate nutrition the human body is powerless to resist health breakdown. Indeed, as was indicated in the second chapter, better housing, coupled with dietary improvements and sanitation, were responsible for the rise in health standards in the eighteenth and nineteenth centuries, rather than the intervention of physicians. Access to basic foodstuffs should be within the means of all individuals, and health professionals thus need to be closely allied with agricultural planners to ensure that nations accept the responsibility to *produce* essential food crops whenever possible. Further, health professionals need to align their work with those involved in food *distribution* to assure that nutritious food reaches people. We need also to educate people to the subtle ways in which the use of technology to make life easier has in fact made it more difficult and less healthy.

We live in a society dominated by technological innovation, and we have created a synthetic environment in which we are surrounded by the artificial products of our technology. Our homes are now commonly built of imitation stone or brick; tiles are made of synthetic slate, and the traditional thatched roofs and fences are even made of fake thatching. We use plastic, glass, or metal tables, set with plastic, glass, or metal dishes - often upon plastic tablecloths. We even manufacture artificial flowers to decorate rooms bathed in artificial light. Carpets, rugs, draperies, upholstery, not to mention our clothes, are predominately made of synthetic fibers. We manufacture and use artificial fireplaces, often replete with simulated logs and a fake hearth to be swept with an 'old-fashioned' synthetic corn broom. New technologies have made it possible to fabricate the whole of nature.

Having accustomed ourselves to our increasingly artificial environment, the development of synthetic foods and the treatment of our water with chemicals represent a logical extension of the artificial world we have already consecrated. Such a world - as 'enriched' as we may think it to be - betrays our alienation from nature, and as we are ourselves a part of nature, the price to be paid is dear.

Nowhere is the cost dearer in health terms than in respect of what we eat and drink. Largely as a result of extensive advertising, we have become conditioned to regard as attractive to the eye and pleasing to the palate a wide array of synthetic and processed foods which not only posses far less nutritive value than the 'real thing,' but also contain chemical substances positively harmful to health. Let us consider a few of these.

> "If a child grows up thinking that the jolly rancher's palate of flavors like cherry and watermelon is what [real] food tastes like...when they taste the real thing, it [will not] taste right... When given a choice between fresh and artificial raspberry flavor, I suspect they might choose the artificial..." Audrey Cross, Associate Professor of Nutrition at the Columbia School of Public Health in 'Do artificial flavors spoil us for the taste of real food', *New York Times*, January 3rd 1996.

In 1972 the new president of a major U.S. food company criticized a detractor for his expose of the company's lemon cream pie which contained no real lemon, no natural cream and, surprisingly, no eggs. The new president defended the product on the grounds that the company "was doing society a real favor by putting artificial ingredients into their pies because this was getting us used to the future when all of our foods will be artificial" (Marshall Elfron, interviewed by Philip Noble, "Uncommon Conversations," *Universal Press Syndicate,* 1972).

The birth of synthetic foods

There is little doubt that modern society and the technology to which it has given birth have radically transformed our lives. While there is much about modern civilization to be applauded, the synthesizing which now characterizes virtually every area of food production is not one of them. Although we have - largely by dint of advertising - come to regard as palatable and attractive the wide array of synthetic foods which have been fabricated as surrogates for real ones, it is clear that the progressive use of synthetic ingredients as partial and in some instances complete substitutes for nature's own products has resulted in a progressive diminution or reduction in the nutritive value of what we eat.

Synthetic foods are edible substances manufactured in a laboratory from a variety of nonfood sources, particularly chemical combinations designed to simulate the natural harvest of field and pasture, orchard and farm, lake, stream, and sea. Meticulous attention is paid to duplicating the taste, texture, and appearance of the real thing, with little or no regard for their nutritional content.

Synthetic fruit

Synthetic fruit, for example, has been around for decades and is widely used in breakfast cereals, fruit cakes, pie fillings, and fruit bars and cookies. One example is the synthetic cherry, fabricated and patented in 1946, and currently marketed in many countries, including France, Italy, Switzerland, Holland, Finland, Australia, and in the U.S., where it is sold commercially in five sizes.

The synthetic cherry is formed by a commercial process in which a chemical solution of sodium alginate (which has been artificially colored and flavored to approximate real cherries) is allowed to drip into a bath of calcium salt such as calcium chloride. The interaction between these chemicals causes a thin covering of insoluble calcium alginate to accumulate on the outside of each drop. The structure formed eventually gels as the calcium ions penetrate progressively towards the centre, and the resulting artificial cherry is uniform in appearance, stable, and unaffected by heat, thus making it especially attractive for commercial baking. [5]

With the decline in the availability of natural raisins, and the increased demand for their use in breads, cakes, muffins, cereals, and the like, raisin-flavored granules have become an attractive alternative to the 'real' thing.' The commercial production of artificial raisins is considerable, as they can be produced in any season, on demand, and at a price much cheaper than genuine raisins can. Among the ingredients of artificial raisins are usually sugar, vegetable oil and fats, corn syrup, preservatives, and raisin flavoring, which itself may be either natural of artificial. Once again, the nutritive value of the product is extremely low, and there is now a vast literature to suggest that several of the ingredients standardly used in the fabrication of artificial fruit and vegetables may be hazardous to health.

Refined sugar

It is estimated that every year Americans consume on average approximately 66 pounds of sugar per person. Indeed, about half our carbohydrates derive from highly refined sugar products such as those provided by processed and synthetic foods. [6, 7] Traditionally, sugar is in fact listed in the class of carbohydrates. In order to see why this can be misleading, it is helpful to remember that the term "sugar" refers to a group of compounds, of which table sugar (sucrose) represents only one member. The sugar in blood, for example, is not *sucrose* but *glucose,* another member of the sugar group, and as such has a different molecular configuration. Although sucrose and glucose may be found in relatively small amounts in virtually all plant foods, the sugar found in natural foods manifests itself primarily as an aggregate of glucose or what is commonly known as a complex carbohydrate.

The human digestive system is particularly adept at assimilating large quantities of complex carbohydrates in the form of starch by breaking down the aggregate or complex of glucose molecules into the individual molecules of which it consists. The complicated physiological process by way of which digestion achieves this in fact contributes to the healthy function of the body, including the digestive process itself. Unrefined sugars in the form of complex carbohydrates contain important quantities of fiber, for example, which assist not only in the *process* of digestion, but in the *effectiveness* of the body to make use of what is digested. There is evidence to suggest, for instance, that the absorption of a range of vitamins and minerals depends on the presence of sufficient fiber in the foods we eat. Simple or refined sugar deprives the body of the fiber which accompanies complex carbohydrates, thus serving to cause disruptions within the established balance of body biochemistry. [8]

Continued biochemical derangements are believed by many researchers to lead to major degradations of body functions such as diabetes, heart disease, hyperactivity and pathological behavior, obesity, and even cancer.

Processed foods and the loss of vitamins and minerals

The consequence of the commercial processing of natural foods is significant. When flour is milled, for example, it loses approximately 80 percent of each of twenty-four known vitamins and minerals. This is one of the main reasons why bread and other products relying on milled flour are *enriched.* Of the twenty-four vitamins and minerals lost, it has been customary to replace only three vitamins and one mineral, since the addition of other nutrients interferes with commercial aspects of the manufacturing process. In any case it is clear that even when the flour is enriched, statements such as "this product contains 60 percent of the RDA of vitamin B, or of vitamin C" are extremely misleading. [9, 10] To think that the nutritive value of processed food can be restored simply by replacing the vitamins and minerals destroyed in the process of manufacturing is sadly naïve. Vitamins can be regarded as links in a chain; once the order of the links or the presence of one or other link is changed, the strength and integrity of the chain as a whole is changed. In other words, the definition of "vitamins" and "minerals" is a matter largely determined by biological function. It is only in the appropriate biological context that a vitamin can function. Once the integrated pattern of the cellular organization of flour has been degraded, the appropriate context of balance within which such vitamins might effectively function is *no longer present.* As in the story of Humpty Dumpty, you might have all the pieces, but that does not mean you can put Humpty together again.

The nutritional degradation of white bread

In the roller-miller process of white flour production, the bran and embryo (germ) contained within the original grain are both removed to ensure that commercial flour is less susceptible to spoilage, since the oil of wheat germ tends to become rancid with prolonged storage. While the bran would otherwise provide a good source of roughage, the discarded embryo is also rich in vitamins and an array of fatty acids which the human body cannot itself manufacture. Indeed, the fatty acids (oil of wheat germ) removed are precisely those the body requires to synthesize nerve tissue, which in turn impacts upon the synchronized functions of the central nervous system.

Even the principal protein of the grain, gluten, is deliberately destroyed or radically altered to accommodate the commercial objectives of the bread industry. It is the gluten which provides the dough with sufficient elasticity to permit the natural process of leavening, as when the dough expands into an airy loaf. The problem is that only the "hard" or best quality grains are possessed of enough gluten content to produce the upstanding loaves to which we have become accustomed. To overcome this difficulty the manufacturers standardly treat the protein of the flour with sodium iodate and potassium bromate, thereby converting the original gluten molecules into a rigid lattice suitable for leavening. By radically altering the structure of the protein, the manufacturer is able to use wheat of lower and often inferior quality to produce flour with consistent baking properties. Once the bran and embryo have been removed, benzoyl peroxide or chlorine is employed in the service of bleaching the flour to the color of alabaster white which characterizes the flour commercially available.

In the interest of increasing the shelf-life of bread and ensuring soft, white, airy loaves, a major portion of the vitamin and mineral content is destroyed. The nutritional impact is subtle but staggering. In its wisdom nature includes with the starch content in flour, the principal component of the grain, the full range of vitamins and minerals essential to the digestion of the starch. The sad truth is that despite attempts to enrich bread, flour which has been bleached and oxidized has been robbed of in excess of twenty essential vitamins and minerals.

The loss of vitamins and minerals through canning and freezing

Flour is not the only natural product which is severely affected by the technology of mass food production. In essence, the commercial process of preserving foods involves either discarding essential components susceptible to spoilage, as in the case of white flour, or adding a poison to prevent the growth of microorganisms. The poison sodium benzoate, for instance, is a common additive to a wide range of commercially bottled products. The human body is thus required to deal with noxious preservatives which retard the process of digestion while also poisoning the body itself.

Although canning and freezing do not rely on the addition of preservatives, the processes involved in the production of canned and frozen food products have a detrimental effect on their vitamin and mineral content. In the case of commercial canning, the application of heat for preserving causes staggering nutritional losses. Lima beans thus preserved, for example, have been shown to lose up to 84% of thiamin, 76% of vitamin C, 72% of pantothenic acid, 67% of riboflavin, 64% of niacin, 62% of folic acid, 55% of vitamin A, and 47% of pyridoxine. [11, 12] It is also well established that a considerable portion of the mineral content of canned vegetables ends up being leached into the water.

Freezing brings about its own peculiar degradation of the nutritional value of fresh foods. It is estimated that approximately one-third of the vitamin C of frozen foods is lost in the initial blanching process. Prolonged periods of frozen storage also contribute to a continuous loss of the vitamins originally contained in the food.

Contamination of food

In addition to the problems associated with processed foods, the mass production of meat from cows, pigs, and chickens signals a further degradation of our health. In the U.S. alone some 76 million cases of food poisoning are reported each year, while many cases go unrecognized. Despite persistent efforts to clean and screen poultry and meats, it is estimated that nearly 40% of all chickens sold on the commercial market in the U.S. are contaminated with salmonella, along with 12% of all pork products and 5% of red meats. [13] When one considers that the sanitary regulations governing the production of foods in the U.S. are tighter than in most other countries, there is genuine cause to worry.

Part of the problem is that we have not yet developed adequate methods for detecting the array of bacterial contaminations caused by the mass production of foods. A larger problem is the modern habit of producing food for mass consumption. In order to promote growth and control disease among farm animals, 70 percent of the antibiotics produced in the United States per annum are used on poultry, pigs and beef cattle. [14] In consequence, an increasing number of cases of food poisoning are being reported in which the bacteria involved are resistant to the antibiotics which might otherwise have been used to treat them in humans.

Pesticides complicate the problem even further, a point we will consider in more detail later in this chapter. Limiting the health risks associated with pesticides solely to their potential to increase the risk of cancer in humans, it is estimated that some 80% of pesticide carcinogens derive from ten chemical compounds applied to fifteen foods, including tomatoes, corn, and grapes. Urethane, linked with cancer, for example, has ever been found in a number of brands of popular wines. According to the National Academy of Sciences in the U.S., at least 98% of the potential risk from pesticide residues on food could be eliminated if the residue levels were rigorously controlled, which sadly they are not. [15]

Water

The year 1990 closed the decade of "International Drinking Water Supply and Sanitation," the target of which was that all people will be provided with a continuous supply of safe drinking water and appropriate means of sanitation. However, this aim is still to be realized, and many infants continue to go on dying from diarrheal diseases, due largely to insufficient commitment and funding in many countries. If two weeks' expenditure on military matters were spent over a year on the provision of clean water, the entire world could be supplied. Having set countless international goals of health for all, national governments must accept that if this aim is to be realized they must allocate sufficient funding to secure the procurement and distribution of safe water.

Water pollution

Proper nutrition could well be said to state with ensuring that you drink enough water. It is recommended that depending upon climate and level of physical activity, the daily intake of water would be somewhere between ten and twelve eight-ounce glasses per day. Humans can survive without food for weeks, but without water human life cannot be sustained after a few days. Among the many health problems caused by not drinking enough water are poor muscle and skin tone, muscle atrophy, joint soreness, post-exercise muscle aches, increased toxicity in the body, kidney stones and, perhaps surprisingly, fluid retention and obesity. Sufficient intake of water contributes to weight control in a number of ways. First, it assists in flushing waste products out of the body, thereby diminishing water retention associated with some forms of bloating. Second, sufficient water figures in the process whereby body fat is metabolized. Third, it may assist in suppressing the appetite, particularly if it is drunk just prior to meals. Since seventy percent of the body consists of water, it is essential not only that we drink enough of it, but that it is as pure as possible. This brings us to the health problems now confronting modern cities which standardly add chemicals to our drinking water, and here we are caught in a dilemma.

Given that one consequence of unbridled technological development is an earth now drenched in acid rain and beleaguered by chemical waste dumps, it is no surprise that we bear witness to the continued poisoning of our oceans, lakes, rivers, and aquifers. The sad truth is that our drinking water needs to be purified, because we have despoiled it. To compensate for the chemical pollution of our water we add more chemicals to it in the hope that technology will make better even those things which by its intervention it is bound to make worse. This is why we standardly 'purify' our drinking water with chlorine, virulent bleach presumed to kill dangerous bacteria. Research has now shown, however, that chlorine is itself a significant health hazard. [16]

Chlorination and health

We have come to accept the presence of chlorine in our drinking water as one of the necessary, though slightly unpleasant aspects of maintaining community health. Somewhere along the way, most of us have learned that a number of contagious diseases such as typhoid and cholera have been virtually eradicated by filtering and chlorinating our municipal water supplies.

1988 marked the century of water chlorination. In 1888 a patent on chlorination of water was granted to Dr Albert R. Leeds, professor of chemistry at Stevens Institute of Technology, Hoboken, New Jersey. Leeds showed that chlorine could be used as the basis of a method of disinfection to control pathogens responsible for waterborne diseases. In the following year the first chlorination of a public water supply was initiated at Adrian, Michigan, though it was not until 1908 that chlorination was introduced on a large scale at the then-huge Boonton Reservoir waterworks in Jersey City, New Jersey. By World War II the practice of chlorination was widely established in the United States. [17]

The potential health risks from chlorinated water

Chlorine is without question a very reactive and poisonous chemical and it would seem ludicrous that such a toxic substance could be deliberately added to public drinking water without carrying out beforehand an extensive study of the possible harmful health effects. There are strong indications that the relevant longitudinal studies were neglected in the case of chlorination. In 1951 Dr. W. J. Llewellyn wrote to the editor of the *Journal of the American Medical Association:*

> What studies have been made to determine the deleterious effects of heavily chlorinated water that is used for drinking purposes? The water supply in our

> town is chlorinated but not filtered. At times it is possible to smell the chlorine. Could this harm the gastrointestinal or the genitourinary tract? [18]

The editor replied:

> A search of the literature did not reveal any organized investigations on the problem of the effect of heavily chlorinated water on the human body. Allergic manifestations of chlorinated water have been reported. Many cases of asthma have been traced to an allergy to chlorinated water. In all these cases the asthma was relieved or disappeared when the patient drank distilled or unchlorinated water. [19]

That same year an awareness of the detrimental health aspects of chlorination was expressed by H. M. Sinclair, Director of the Laboratory for Human Nutrition, Oxford University.

Commenting on heart disease, Sinclair raised what in those times must have seemed an almost incredible accusation. He wrote: "It is possible that one of the greatest public health measures ever introduced - the chlorination of public water supply - could assist [heart] disease." [20] Sinclair himself could hardly have perceived how prophetic the alleged association would be between chlorination and heart disease. In a suggestive study by Ronald Pataki, an astounding correlation of just these factors was discovered in Jersey City, the place where the first comprehensive chlorination of municipal water supplies began eighty years ago. Pataki found that the severity of heart disease among people over fifty years of age correlated directly with the quantities of chlorinated tap water they were accustomed to drinking. Interestingly, he also found a statistically significant correlation which showed that those people over fifty who did *not* suffer from heart disease standardly drank mostly nonchlorinated fluids, bottled water, or boiled water (it is known that chlorine can be released as a gas from water which is boiled). [21]

Passwater reports that in South India the water is chlorinated, while in North India it is not, and consistent with Sinclair's original intuition, the incident of heart disease in the South is considerably higher than in the North. He also points out that since the drinking water of the northern capital city, New Delhi, has been chlorinated, the heart-disease rate of that city has, sadly, begun to climb. [22] In the *National Enquirer* (December 24th, 1974) Dr. Joseph Price of Saginaw General Hospital in Michigan is quoted as saying:

> Chlorine is the cause of an unprecedented disease epidemic which includes heart attacks and strokes. Chlorine is an insidious poison. Most medical researchers were led to believe it was safe, but we are now learning the hard way that all the time we thought we were preventing epidemics of one disease, we were creating another. Two decades after the start of chlorinating our drinking water in 1904, the present epidemic of heart trouble and cancer began. [23]

In his book *Coronaries, Cholesterol, Chlorine,* Price reports a study in which, in contract to the control group, chickens reared on chlorinated water *all* showed evidence of either atherosclerosis of the aorta or obstruction of the circulatory system. [24] Chlorine is further implicated in heart disease by the work of E. P. Benditt, Professor in the Department of Pathology at the University of Washington, whose research in 1974 associated plaque formation in the arteries with chlorination. His research suggested that because of mutations in their genetic program caused by mutagenic or even carcinogenic substances in the bloodstream, and other substances released by the arteries as a result of high blood pressure, cells in the arterial wall proliferate to form plaque.[25]

Studies by Revis et al. add further strength to the insidious link between water chlorination and heart disease. They report that they observed "hypercholesterolemia and cardiac hypertrophy in pigeons and rabbits exposed to chlorinated drinking water" [26] and "significant increases in plasma cholesterol and aortic atherosclerosis in pigeons exposed to three commonly used drinking water disinfectants" - chlorine, chlorine dioxide and monochloramine. [27]

In the mid-seventies the issue of the health hazards associated with chlorinated water was raised from yet another perspective. Awareness of increasing levels of toxic chemicals in water, particularly chlorine containing organic compounds, prompted the Environmental Protective Agency (EPA) to undertake a national survey to determine the quality of drinking water throughout the U.S. Of particular concern was the formation of chloroform resulting from the use of chlorine for water purification. In 1975 the results of the survey were published, and revealed that *drinking water from all the 79 cities tested contained some amount of the suspected carcinogen chloroform.* [28] Concentrations of chloroform varied from less than 1.0 pp in Strasburg, Pennsylvania, to 311 pp in Miami, Florida. Despite these astonishing results, the EPA representative assured the press that the American people should not react with any sense of panic. Although mores than 240,000 sizable drinking-water supply systems in the U.S. were deemed likely to be contaminated with one or more or six toxic chemicals, at least two of which are suspected carcinogens, the representatives warned against any overreaction to the findings of the survey, saying that "the benefits of using chlorine far outweigh the potential health risks from chlorine-derived organic compounds." [29] Despite these assurances, it is clear that the health hazards associated with the presence in drinking water of chlorination-induced chemicals are of the utmost seriousness. In 1975 in New Orleans, Louisiana, the tap water was found to contain more organic chlorine compounds that untreated Mississippi River water. [30] The EPA's assurances seemed less convincing when in the following year a major research study reported a statistical correlation between the incidence of cancer among the New Orleans population and their municipal water supplies.[31]

By 1987 a number of studies documented the wide range of toxic substances in drinking water which derive from chlorination. [32] In 1987 a study undertaken by M. K. Smith et. al. demonstrated that a number of the chlorine-induced components found in drinking water have in laboratory animals caused reduced fertility and increased failure of early implantation. The birth weight of the pups was reduced significantly and the prenatal survival of the pups was adversely affected by at least two of the halogenated compounds. Short-term tests for the carcinogenic affects of several of the chlorinated compounds also proved positive, thereby reinforcing earlier findings which linked chlorination and cancer. [33, 34, 35]

Fluoridation and the politics of health

The introduction of the fluoridation provides a good example not only of the health risks associated with the addition of chemicals to our water, but of the potential influence of politics and vested interests in the determination of health politics. [36]

In small amounts (one part per million) soluble fluorides have been alleged to produce beneficial affects on the teeth of growing children, though they are admitted to have no such effects on the teeth of adults. Whatever their success in the reduction of dental decay, it is important to be mindful that fluoride is itself a powerful poison which - whether we like the idea or not - is automatically added to the municipal drinking waters of many countries around the globe.

The notion of "mass-medicating" the public with such a highly toxic substance as fluoride becomes all the more worrying when we discover that for nearly four decades fluorides were standardly used as a rat and cockroach poison. Equally disconcerting is the fact that the chemical warfare "nerve gases" (esters of fluophosphoric acids) still in use in some parts of the world are among the more important organic fluorine derivatives. We know that fluoride effluents from industry have also caused untold losses to crops and livestock around the world, so it is easy to appreciate the grave concern on the part of some that the government approves the compulsory ingestion of a poison to obtain partial control of what is conventionally regarded as a noncommunicable disease (i.e., tooth decay). How it is then that fluoridation has come to be hailed by others as a major contribution to the advancement of community health?

Health policy decisions and vested interests

The fluoridation controversy becomes especially intriguing when we realize that fluorine wastes from industry have figured for nearly a century as one of the main pollutants of our lakes, streams, and aquifers. The aluminium industry in particular has been implicated in environmental fluoride contamination, as sodium aluminium fluoride features as an essential element in the production of aluminium by electrolysis. Historically, fluoride has been regarded as a toxic substance to be kept out of the environment - the problem for industry has always been how to dispose of it without destroying the environment. Imagine then how attractive the idea would be to aluminium manufacturers if it could be shown that one of the beneficial side-effects of minimal dental fluorosis (fluoride poisoning of the teeth) is that the enamel surface of the tooth is hardened somewhat to reduce the incidence of dental decay. Imagine the joy of aluminium manufacturers if rather than having to pay to dispose of fluoride contaminants, *they were paid to supply them to fluoridate the drinking waters of the world.*

It happens that the history of the fluoridation program betrays a remarkable series of fortuitous coincidences of just this kind, along with a number of intriguing connections between the public health bodies responsible for the introduction of fluoridation and the aluminium industry. In the late 1930s the United States Public Health Service (PHS) was sponsored under the Department of the Treasury, the chief officer of which was then Andrew Mellon, who coincidentally also happened to be the owner of the Aluminium Corporation of America (ALCOA). In 1939 *The Mellon Institute* (established and controlled by the family of Andrew Mellon), employed a scientist, Dr. Gerald Cox, to find a viable market for the industrial fluoride wastes associated with the production of aluminium. Of this intriguing series of connections between the interests of ALCOA and the introduction of fluoridation Dennis Stevenson writes cynically:

> Dr. Cox then proposed artificial water fluoridation as a means of reducing tooth decay. What better way to solve the huge and costly problem of disposing of toxic waste from Aluminium manufacture than getting paid to put it in the drinking water? What an incredible coincidence - ALCOA and the original fluoridation proposal. [37]

Nor does the chain of seeming coincidences end here.

Caldwell refers to the very interesting testimony of Florence Birmingham on May 25, 26, 27, 1954 before the Committee on Interstate and Foreign Commerce, which had organized a series of hearings on the fluoridation issue. As President of the Massachusetts Women's Political club, Miss Birmingham was on the occasion representing some fifty thousand women. She is recorded as saying:

> In 1944 Oscar Ewing was put on the payroll of the Aluminium Company of America, as attorney; at an annual salary of $750,000. This fact was established at a Senate hearing and became part of the Congressional record. Since the Aluminium Company had no big litigation pending at the time, the question might logically be asked, why such a large fee? A few months later Mr. Ewing was made Federal Security Administrator with the announcement that he taking a big salary cut in order to serve his country. As head of the Federal Security Agency (now the Department of Health, Education, and Welfare), he immediately started the ball rolling to sell "rat poison" by the ton instead of in dime packages. . . .The Aluminium Company of America then began selling sodium fluoride tablets to put in the drinking water." [38]

The series of events which thereafter led to the apparently inevitable implementation of fluoridation deserve to be reviewed. In 1945 Grand Rapids, Michigan, was selected as the site of the first major longitudinal study of the effects of fluoridation on the public at large. Comparisons were to be made with the city of Muskegon, Michigan, which remained unfluoridated so that it could be used as a control. Although the experiment was supposed to be undertaken over the course of ten years to determine any cumulative side-effects which might result from the fluoridation of municipal water, Ewing intervened after only five years to declare the success of the study in showing fluoridation to be safe. As Walker puts it: "In June 1950 half-way through the experiment, the U.S. / P.H.S. under its Chief, Oscar Ewing, "endorsed" the safety and effectiveness of artificial fluoridation; and encouraged its immediate adoption through the States." [39]

One year later Ewing was able to convince the American Congress that fluoridation was a necessity, and a total of two million dollars (an enormous sum of money in those days) was immediately directed to promote the fluoridation program throughout the U.S.A. [40]

Mandatory medication by fluoridation was not of course peculiar to the United States. Australians have for more than five decades been subjected to forced fluoridation of their drinking water. In 1953 the National Health and Medical Research Council of Australia lent its support to the mandatory mass-medication of Australians. [41] Today, Australia has 'distinguished' itself by promoting a fluoridation program with such vigor that Australia now ranks as the most comprehensively fluoridated country in the world. For example, by 2012 Queensland health aims for 90 percent of the drinking water in Queensland, Australia, to be fluoridated. [42]

Can fluoridation be kept at safe levels?

Although 1 ppm is standardly defined as that level of fluoride concentration which provides maximal protection against dental decay, with minimal clinically observable dental fluorosis, controversy ranges widely as to adverse effects of prolonged fluoride exposure even at this level. As early as 1942, it was reported that in areas of endemic fluorosis with fluoride concentrations of 1ppm or less, children with poor nutrition suffered skeletal defects, coupled with severe mottling of teeth.

Even if one grants that fluoride concentrations of 1ppm are relatively safe, it has become increasingly clear that individual levels of *safe* fluoride ingestion cannot be adequately controlled. Drinking-water dosages of fluoride, for example, will depend partly on variable factors such as thirst. Liquid intakes also vary according to age, work situation, climate and season, and levels of exercise. Athletes, for instance, tend to consume more water than their nonathletic counterparts. Adjustments to municipal water supplies cannot accommodate satisfactorily the wide array of relevant individual differences of this kind.

In addition fluorides are ingested in varying quantities from many unsuspected sources. Fluoride tablets, seemingly innocuous mouth-washes, gels, and even water-based tablets contribute to dangerous increases in fluoride levels well beyond the recommended 1 ppm contained in drinking water. Although the point has yet to be established definitively, it has been suggested that aluminium cooking utensils and non-stick cookware which are coated with Tetrafluoroethylene are inclined to exude fluoride into food, particularly if they have surface scratches or are overheated. [43, 44]

By far the most common source of additional fluoride ingestion beyond the accepted 1 ppm in drinking water, however, comes from beverage consumption. Beverages which contain fluorinated water include reconstituted juices, punches, popsicles, water-based frozen deserts, carbonated beverages, and even beer. It has now been shown that prolonged exposure to fluorides may actually increase rather than diminish the incidence of tooth decay. Enzymatic damage related to enamel mineralization creates a parotic tooth far more susceptible of caries than would otherwise be the case. [45]

In a major study on the adverse effects of fluoridation Bassin reported in 2001 that there is a 'significant link between fluoridated drinking water and osteosarcoma, a rare and often fatal bone cancer in boys'. [46] This study helped to confirm previous studies by Dr Perry Cohn, New Jersey Health Department, who found 'higher rates of osteosarcoma among boys in fluoridated areas than those in non-fluoridated areas'. [47]

The politics of health

The controversy surrounding fluoridation raises a number of important socio-ethical issues which cannot be overlooked. One of the most burning questions is whether the fluoridation program represents a milestone in the advancement of community health or the opportunistic outcome of a powerful lobby concerned largely to advance its own vested interests at the expense of the interests of the public. The potential and actual health risks associated with fluoridation have not been sufficiently appreciated by those in favor of fluoridation. The intentional introduction of fluorides in drinking water has certainly not received the rigorous scrutiny and testing *properly brought to bear* on the wide array of available medical drugs, many of which can be bought without prescription. Even if it were granted that the addition of a minimal amount of fluoride to our water supply was both safe and effective in the reduction of caries in the teeth of children, the relevant dosage of fluorides could not be satisfactorily restricted to ensure that the harmful effects of fluoride did not outweigh the alleged beneficial effects. Well-intentioned or not, it is manifestly clear that the partial prevention of dental decay is not the bottom line of the fluoridation debate when the panacea has become the poison.

Insecticides and Pesticides

In January 1940, Sir Albert Howard wrote in the preface of his seminal work *An Agricultural Testamount:*

> "Since the Industrial Revolution the processes of growth have been speeded up to produce the food and raw materials needed by the population and the factory. Nothing effective has been done to replace the loss of fertility involved in this vast increase in crop and animal production. The consequences have been disastrous. Agriculture has become unbalanced: the land is in revolt; diseases of all kinds are on the increase; in many parts of the world Nature is removing the worn out soil by means of erosion." [48]

Howard goes on to argue in his book that the use of inorganic fertilizers together with excessive irrigation and over-cultivation are destroying the fertility of the soil, and that as a consequence there is increased disease in plants, animals and man.

The over-cultivation and over-irrigation of the soil gradually occurred as agricultural progress came to be defined in terms of increased yield per hectare. The development of machines to convert concentrated energy to mechanical power gave a whole new sense to the concept of efficiency. Efficiency, the watchword of the mechanical paradigm and the Industrial Revolution, was carried into the realm of agriculture. Machines were increasingly used to divert and pump water in vast quantities and to cultivate the soil on a scale never before possible.

Liebig's observations of the increased growth of plants which occurred when phosphates were mixed with soil, led to a proliferation of plant chemical whose specific purpose was to increase the soil crop yield per hectare. One such example was the use of sulfuric acid to increase the solubility of phosphates patented by J.B. Lawes in 1842.[49] This form of phosphate later became known as superphosphate . Within a few years, increasing quantities of potassium salts, from deposits at Stassfurt in Germany, and nitrate salts from Chile, were being transported to various parts of the world.

Given this worldwide dissemination of superphosphates the compositions of soil was rapidly altered on a worldwide basis. Fertilizers containing a mixture of nitrogen, phosphorus and potassium compounds became known as 'complete' fertilizers, [50] reinforcing and entrenching in the minds of farmers the misleading NPK mentality. As research on the chemical control of plants continued, agricultural scientists discovered that individual types of crops were found to respond to particular ratios of NPK fertilizer mixes. For example, the ration for potatoes was 4:8:10, for wheat 2:12:6, clover 0:12:15, and strawberries 5:8:7. These differing fertilizers requirements, together with the development of particular cultivation configurations of farm machinery for different crops, led to the practice of cultivating ever-larger areas of land for a single type of crop. Monoculturing was thus incorporated as part of the all-pervasive western perspective devoted to growth and efficiency. F. Gramham comments:

> "By the end of World War II, farming had evolved from a way of life to an industry. The farmer acquired the approach and the philosophy of the manufacturer. The small family farm, which once produced a variety of fruits, vegetables, and diary foods, now merged with a dozen of its fellows to form a single vast 'factory farm' producing a single crop. In the interests of economy, every move was directed, every machine was adapted, to plant, nourish, and harvest that crop – whether it was celery, apples, corn, or soy beans. A new word – monoculture – found a place in the dictionary."[51]

Biodiversity is a life-supporting characteristic of nature. Since the production of modern farming the genetic diversity of our agricultural plants has been rapidly vanishing. This century, the United States has lost more than 90 per cent of its 20,000 varieties of agricultural plants. Since 1930, 80 per cent of the varieties of maize in Mexico have been lost and China now only grows 1000 strains of wheat, compared with 10,000 or so strains it grew before 1949. This decline in agricultural biodiversity is leaving our crops prone to pest and plague. [52]

Monoculture is a distortion of nature which, in a sense, produces a 'plague' of plants. What was missed in the equation was that this extreme ecology inevitability results in a plague of insects. Given the commitment to technology as the panacea of all ills, chemical controls or pesticides were quickly enlisted in the battle against the armies of invading insects. It is revealing that the rapid growth of monoculture after World War II, which was paralleled by an inordinate expansion in farm machinery and fertilizer sales, was also accompanied by an expanding use of pesticides. [53] What is even more apocalyptic is the evidence which establishes that concomitant with the growth of technological farming, the percentage of crops lost to pests and disease increased accordingly.

Giving evidence in 1951 before the Delaney Committee inquiry into pesticide use in the United States, R.L. Webster described how, in 1909, only single sprayings of arsenate were used each year. By 1926, pests had become so much more troublesome, that five or six additional sprayings were required during the season. He went on to say:

> Worm control in the Pacific North-west was becoming more difficult, year by year. We now know that the codling moth was acquiring a degree of resistance...More and more lead arsenate was used every year and at one time Washington State was using 25 per cent of the entire production in the United States. The peak came in 1943, when more than 17,000,000 pound (lbs) were sold in the state.[54]

Webster's observations contrast revealingly with those of Howard. Howard had reported that of the crops grown in humus-rich soil around 500,000 villages in India, suffered remarkably little from pests. [55] He also had argued that the replacement of animal manure and compost by artificial NPK fertilizers was directly linked to the increased susceptibility of plants to disease and insect attack.

With the spread of artificials and the exhaustion of the original supplies of humus, there has been a corresponding increase in the diseases of crops and of the animals which feed on them. If the spread of foot-and-mouth disease in Europe and its comparative insignificance among well-fed animals in the East are compared, or if the comparison is made between certain areas in Europe, the conclusion is inevitable that there must be an intimate connection between faulty methods of agriculture and animal disease. In crops like potatoes and fruit, the use of the poison spray has closely followed the reduction in the supplies of farmyard manure and the diminution of fertility.[56]

As nature revolted against the mechanical and chemical transformations of the environment, an extensive arsenal of poisons was developed to subdue the revolt. In 1939, P.Muller discovered the insecticide properties of DDT, a chlorinated organic compound first synthesized 65 years earlier. Since that time there has been an exponential increase in the number of synthetic insecticides, herbicides and fungicides available. [57] In 1986, some 1500 active pesticide ingredients were registered in the United States [58] with about 360,000,000 kilograms of these chemicals being applied annually in the agricultural sector alone.[59]

The link between monoculture, fertilizer requirements and pesticide use is well illustrated by the farming of corn in the United States. This single crop consumed 44 per cent of the total United States fertilizer use, with the application rate being as high as 340 kilograms per hectare. [60] At the same time, to control insect attack a massive 43 per cent of the total pesticides used in the United States were applied to this same crop. [61] Despite this huge application of poisonous pesticides in the name of technological progress, R. Nade points out that the percentage of pre-harvest crops lost to insect damage increased from 9 per cent in 1945 to 12 per cent in 1989. [62] This is due, in part, to the increasing resistance of many pests to pesticides [63] and also possibly to a decreased immunity of plants to pests, which Howard suggests is a consequence of the use of chemical fertilizers.

There is a mordant irony in the fact that in India, where in the 1930's crops grown on fertile soils suffered remarkably little from pests, the emphasis on economic growth and chemical technology has led to a tenfold increase in pesticide consumption during the past two decades. Motivated by the technological imperative, India in 1990-91, consumed an estimated one million tonnes of pesticides. [64]

Howard also noted that plants grown for food on fertile soil, free of chemical fertilizers but rich in humus, confer upon the animals and humans which eat them the health benefit of increased immunity to disease. [65] Among the many examples of communities whose immune functions have been improved, Howard cites the Hunzas in Pakistan. The health, beauty, fitness and longevity of these people has provided discussion topics in numerous articles in the popular media. [66] It was not until 1963, however, that medical research began to confirm certain of the claims which figured in these popular reports.[67]

Recent findings have added further support to Howard's claims for compost-grown food. D. Pitt and co-workers at Exeter University found that garden compost can suppress economically significant plant diseases by between 60 and 80 per cent, and can sometimes eliminate them altogether. It was found, for instance, that an 80 per cent reduction in the disease 'take all' in wheat, could be achieved using compost, while red core in strawberries was reduced by 90 per cent. Club root in cabbage was eliminated completely. It appears that organisms in the compost suppress the growth of disease-causing bacteria and fungi. [68]

The adverse effects of the worldwide use of chemical fertilizers for the health of the world's inhabitants are still only being recognized. For instance, the high-yield rice, wheat and maize varieties of the 'Green Revolution' which depend on the liberal use of inorganic fertilizers, are usually low in minerals and vitamins. Because these new 'technology' crops have displaced local foods, the diet of many people in the developing world is now dangerously low in iron, zinc and vitamin A, and other micronutrients.[69]

The extent to which artificial fertilizers undermine the microbial fungal ecosystems of soil is still not adequately appreciated, though research in the area has established a connection between chemical fertilizers and soil erosion.[70] In 1950, J. Russell Smith, Emeritus Professor of Economic Geography at Columbia University, warned that modern crop-based agriculture, such as that used in the production of corn, cotton and tobacco, was not only destroying soil fertility but was, in addition, contributing substantially to soil erosion. He argued urgently for the need to develop a sustainable 'permanent agriculture' to reduce these problems. He made some startling comparisons. The average annual yield of corn in the Appalachian Mountains was 500 kilograms per acre. The yield of chestnut orchards in the mountains of Europe is approximately the same. The chestnuts, however, yield year in and year out for centuries. Corn 'burns out' soil rapidly. Yet the food value and palatability of the chestnut to livestock are comparable to that of corn.[71] Hundreds of other tree crops could be employed by American farmers for producing food for livestock and humans. Unfortunately little attention has been paid to Smith's suggestions. In the meantime, the rapid depletion of natural soil conditioners such as humus fungi, bacteria, earthworms and insects - all of which have in recent years been displaced largely by chemical fertilizers and poisonous sprays - has, according to the technological view, necessitated additional mechanical tilling to achieve soil fertility. However, this additional technological intervention has, in turn, modified the physical structure of the soil, as well as its surface profile and has resulted in increased erosion by wind and rain. Soil erosion is now a major threat to crop production around the world, with a loss of some 80 billion tones of topsoil every year. This is the total amount of topsoil which underlies the whole of Australia's wheatlands.[72]

Farm chemicals have also become a major source of environmental pollution.[73] The application of nitrate fertilizers is a case in point. In the early 1990's F. Haber and C. Bosch developed a process by which nitrogen from the atmosphere could be synthesized with hydrogen (produced by reacting steam with red hot coke) to form ammonia. Since ammonia could be easily oxidized to nitric acid for fertilizer production, the Haber operation conveniently enabled the commercial industry to tap the huge reservoir of nitrogen in the atmosphere. Clever as this sounds, the problem is that the process bypasses nature's own bacteria-moderated nitrogen-fixation processes in the soil itself, which protect the soil from nitrogen saturation.

Huge quantities of nitrogen fertilizers are now applied to the soil around the world each year to promote plant growth. In the United States in 1985, for example, 11 million tonnes of nitrogen were applied to the soil in the form of fertilizers.[74] Once again, this massive manipulation of the natural environment has not been without adverse effects. Nitrate pollution of groundwater and drinking water, for instance, is now a major problem in many countries.[75]

Excessive nitrate levels in vegetables and plants has also become a problem. Attempts have been made to develop varieties of plants with low nitrate accumulation rates in the hope of reducing the health risk of nitrogen poisoning. Nitrates are converted by bacteria in the body to transport oxygen. Excessive nitrogen intake can thus result in a condition of the blood known as methaemoglobinaemia.[76]

Another possible health aspect of the application of nitrate fertilizers to our soils involves an indirect contribution of the greenhouse effect. P.A. Steudler and co-workers have reported that the application of nitrogen fertilizers may reduce the capacity of the soil to act as a sink or absorption table for methane gas. This being so, nitrate fertilizers may actually inhibit the subtle mechanisms in the soil which assist in regulating the atmospheric levels of this naturally produced greenhouse gas.

Since highly soluble chemical fertilizers such as nitrates leach from the soil, they enter the waterways and seas producing a new and inharmonious ecological mix. In some areas, particularly in the North Sea, this new mix has encouraged the phenomenal growth of algae. When the algae die, the biomass is often so large that the bacteria breaking down the dead algae consume all the oxygen in the water, thereby causing fish and other species to suffocate.

Other research has shown that algae give off a sulfur-containing chemical, dimethyl sulfide, which oxidizes in air to form sulfur dioxide, the principle cause of acid rain. It has been estimated that in summer, 25 per cent of the acid rain falling over Europe now comes from huge algae masses in the north sea.[77] This observation illustrates the difficulty in anticipating the extent of environmental disruption and degradation caused by technological intervention. Given the inter-connectivity and delicate relationships which we now know characterize nature, the more intensive the technology, the more it is bound to impact synergistically across the network of these relationships.

Our technologized lifestyle and the exercise / health connection

In recent years there has emerged an increased awareness of the role which exercise can play in helping us to live happier, healthier, and longer lives, and we believe that this aspect of our lifestyle is an important educational component in wholistic health. In the United States one of the nation's largest insurance companies, for example, has in previous years offered discounts of up to 35 percent of the annual premium on life insurance for those policy-holders who engage in accredited exercise programs of thirty or more minutes, three times per week. For those willing to exercise for at least one hour per session five times a week, the discount on premiums is reduced even further. [78] Setting aside incentives of the financial kind, there are many people who regard exercise as so important to health that they would no more go a day without exercising that they would go a day without eating.

What is it about exercise that makes it so essential in the maintenance and promotion of health? Exercise in itself is simply one of a number of factors which contribute to human well-being. To use exercise as a prophylactic against an unhealthy lifestyle is thus self-defeating. The health benefits associated with exercise are minimized for those who systematically abuse themselves through smoking, too little rest, poor eating habits, and excesses of alcohol. Exercise is not a panacea for self-neglect. The aim must be to incorporate exercise into a lifestyle which respects the integrity of the whole person and the many dimensions of personhood which affect health.

The historical connection

In historical terms exercise has figured as a silent component in our evolutionary development. The lifestyle of primitive man, that is to say, was a life of intense physical activity, and it was the strongest, fittest, and cleverest individuals who won the battle for survival. It is generally agreed that the emergence of *homo sapiens* occurred throughout the geological period known as the Pleistocene or Glacial epoch, an interval of approximately one million years. Virtually half of this period was characterized climatically by a succession of glaciations in which much of the earth was covered by ice sheets and glaciers. Life must have been almost unimaginably harsh. Paleolithic (or Old Stone Age) cultural developments during this period amounted to little more than cave-dwelling and the manufacturing of modest stone implements. For virtually the whole of the Glacial epoch our ancestors lived as food-gatherers, depending for subsistence on hunting wild animals, birds, and fish, or gathering nuts, berries, and wild fruits when they could be found. Not only did primitive man have to hunt to survive, but to survive he had to avoid being hunted. Savage animals provided a source of food for him, but he also provided a source of food for them. Most of his time was thus taken up hunting and gathering, or avoiding being hunted and gathered. In such adverse conditions, there is no doubt that exercise played a crucial role in the life of primitive man. In short, he did a lot of running, walking, and fighting; indeed he was constantly fighting for his life.

Our biological inheritance thereby incorporated exercise or intense physical activity in the service of survival, and some of these survival mechanisms such as the "fright-take-flight" kind still dominate our fundamental and instinctual responses. Our contemporary and more sedate, if not sedentary lifestyle, however, no longer provides an outlet for the physical activity which has been so integral a part of our sociocultural evolution. [79] The cholesterol problem we now face in health terms can at least partly be explained by this change of lifestyle. It has been suggested, for example, that the release of cholesterol in the bloodstream was functional when our ancestors were hunting large animals with primitive weapons. Given the likelihood that the animal would be wounded but not initially killed, the hunter would have to follow the animal until it dropped, and this could involve the hunter having to walk for literally days on end without food or rest. In today's society high-pressure jobs give rise to anxiety and stress which seem similarly to simulate the release of cholesterol into the bloodstream but without the concomitant expenditure of physical activity which would in primitive times otherwise have utilized the cholesterol available. [80]

Whether this theory on cholesterol is accepted or not, it should be clear that given our sedentary lifestyle we are generally getting less exercise than our evolutionary development has over the course of nearly a million years led our bodies to expect. But what is the expectation of the body in physiological terms? What happens physiologically when we exercise? Exercise physiology is an enormously complex subject area, and in order to keep this chapter within manageable bounds we will in what follows examine only a few of the basic physiological aspects of exercise.

Exercise and the heart

Inasmuch as exercise affects the heart, it in turn affects the whole circulatory system and thus in some way impacts upon all of the seventy-five trillion cells in the body. Let us first consider how exercise does affect the heart. Put simply, the function of the heart is to pump blood, thereby supplying oxygen and nutrients to the cells, while removing their waste products. On average the resting heart rate for adult males is about 70 beats per minute; for women between 75-80 beats per minute. The heart is itself a muscle, and with sensible exercise the heart muscle grows stronger and becomes a more effective pump. As the strength of the contraction is improved, stroke volume is increased, thus decreasing the number of beats per minute required for the heart to pump the same volume of blood. In consequence, the heart is no longer working as hard to do its job. Since every heartbeat is a muscle contraction, the only chance the heart gets to rest is between beats. The stronger the heart, then, the more chance it gets to rest. Not only will the beat of the heart muscle remain lower at rest, it will also rise more slowly and work less hard to accommodate the blood supply demands of vigorous physical activity.

The ballet of breathing

Exercise can also serve to improve cardiovascular fitness. We have already observed that the heartbeat elevates during exercise to deliver a sufficient supply of blood to the specific muscle groups which require more oxygen. The requirement for more oxygen stimulates breathing, thus allowing the lungs to supply the blood with more oxygen. During this process the tidal flow of air (inhalation-exhalation cycle) per minute is increased from about six liters of air at rest to more that forty-five liters during intense exercise. The lungs may be called upon to oxygenate the blood by more than twenty times its normal resting requirement. During vigorous exercise the demand for additional oxygen is - as we have seen - met by breathing faster and more deeply. These ventilation modifications are for the most part controlled by the involuntary reflex center in the medulla responsible for respiration. The center contains neurons which during inhalation stimulate contractions of the external intercostals muscles (between the ribs) and the muscle of the diaphragm. During exhalation other neurons activate the internal intercostals and diaphragm, thereby completing the oscillating character of the breathing process. Stretch receptors in the lungs monitor the cyclic changes of volume in the thoracic cavity and assist in governing the actual rate of oscillation. The level of carbon dioxide in arterial blood is perhaps the single most important factor in the remarkable coordination of the respiratory impulses, as the rate of breathing increases proportionally to the concentration of carbon dioxide in the blood. [81]

Exercise and bone density

There is some evidence to suggest also that nerve centers in the joints - stimulated by exercise - signal the relevant center of the brain responsible for breathing, muscular coordination, and even bone regeneration. In addition to supporting the body, for example, muscles move bones close to each other through the process we call contraction. As muscles grow stronger, the force they exert on bones through contraction is also greater. This being so, more calcium is deposited in the bones to make them strong enough to accommodate the increased force of muscle contraction. This is why exercise is so important in the rehabilitation process of broken bones and other skeletal deformations.

The "Training Effect"

When bodily processes respond to exercise by making the kind of cardiovascular, skeletal, and neuromuscular changes to which we have been alluding, the process is called the "training effect." [82] Different exercises stimulate different training effects. The principle of Specific Adaption to Imposed Demands (SAID) states that these different training effects can be physiologically classified. Aerobic exercise, for example, brings about a specific adaption, being particularly well suited to improve cardiovascular fitness, endurance, and flexibility. The word "aerobic" means *with air* and refers to moderate-intensity and sustained exercise which requires the body to use large but not intolerably large quantities of oxygen.

Because the quantity of oxygen demanded by the muscle cells is not overwhelming, the aerobic exercise can be performed for protracted periods, thus making the heart grow stronger, improving the capacity of the lungs to process more air with less effort, and increasing the blood supply to the muscles. Aerobic activity not only stimulates a specific cardiovascular adaption, it also speeds up metabolism during the exercise session and for several hours subsequent to the session, thereby assisting weight reduction by ensuring that calories taken into the body are more readily burned.

Exercise and the prevention of heart attack

Implicit in the foregoing discussion have been the intimations of the relevance of exercise for good health, and the time has now come to make at least some of these points explicit. Some form of cardiovascular disease affects 60 million Americans or about 20 percent of the entire population. [83]

Approximately ninety-five percent of all heart attacks result from hardening of the arteries. It is now established that exercise and particularly a circuit-type of weight training can significantly benefit the cardio-respiratory system. Researchers at the Oregon Health Sciences University in the U.S. have shown that with a group of previously untrained men and women, weight training over a period of four months brought about a reduction of 16.5% in LDL cholesterol (low-density lipoprotein cholesterol, a significant factor in hardening of the arteries). In the same study it was also shown that weight training caused an increase of 6.5% in the levels of HDL (high-density lipoprotein cholesterol, which actually reduces the chances of atherosclerosis, thus assisting in the prevention of heart attacks). [84]

In addition to the prevention of heart attack, exercise is now known to lower death rates in respect of a variety of other diseases. In a relevant study undertaken by Dr. Ralph Paffenbarger Jr. et. al. at Stanford University, it has been demonstrated that of 17,000 men, aged between 34-74 years, death rates were one-quarter to one-half lower in those whose weekly exercise regime expended at least 2,000 calories. Death rates were further reduced by those whose calorie expenditure through exercise was around 3,500. [85, 86]

How exercise and diet help prevent cancer

In recent years many people have come to think of AIDS as the leading epidemic of our times. Although AIDS has reached epidemic proportions, it pales in comparison to the ever-increasing incidence of cancer. In the U.S. as of 2006, for example, the *total* number of AIDS cases reported was 56,300, while the number of associated deaths was 14627.87 Comparing the cancer statistics for the year 2005 *alone,* we find that a staggering 1,500,000 *new* cases of cancer were recorded, with an equally staggering 559,312 cancer-associated deaths. [88] Interestingly, both AIDS and cancer result from deficiencies of the immune system, and there is a growing body of literature to suggest that both diseases can be prevented. Exercise and diet are two important preventative measures. To understand just how important, let is first look more closely at what cancer is.

Understanding how cancer works

Although there are more than a hundred different types of cancer, they all involve a certain kind of cell pathology in which an abnormal and unbridled division of cells (e.g., a malignant tumor) spreads throughout the body by invading and destroying otherwise normal cells. The process by which cancer cells spread throughout the body is called *metastasis.* Metastasis relies upon either the bloodstream or the lymphatic system to ensure that cancer cells make their way to parts of the body remote from the original cancer site. This is why primary and secondary tumors are often found at considerable distances from each other.

The wide array of different kinds of cancer is often broken down into two subdivisions (i.e. *carcinomas and sarcomas),* defined by the type of tissue affected by the cancer. [89] "Carcinoma" refers to cancer involving the epithelial tissue which lines the skin and internal organs of the body, and "sarcoma" refers to cancer arising from connective tissues involving bone, cartilage, and the like. Exactly how cancer starts and is spread to these areas remains a matter of controversy, though there is a reasonably clear consensus that the actual process involves two stages: *initiation* and *promotion.* Initiation occurs when the components responsible for cellular reproduction are damaged seemingly irreversibly. Normally, cells within the body are constantly regenerating themselves. For example, the cells within the stomach lining are replaced weekly, the cells of the lungs are regenerated every month, and even the cells of the liver are completely regenerated every six weeks. Appreciation of this point makes it easier to see why damage to the reproductive mechanisms of the cells can cause almost immediate and extensive disruption. "Promotion" refers to the rapid division of the "initiated" or damaged cell. Because the cell is abnormal, its apparently uncontrolled reproduction can quickly and adversely affect the established biochemical harmony of the body.

Cancer and the immune system

There is growing evidence to suggest that many factors such as environmental pollution may initiate cellular abnormalities. To some extent the body can cope with certain of these cellular dysfunctions through an effective system of immune responses which impede the promotion of the cancer by preventing its spread beyond the original site. Exposure to a cancer-causing substance such as asbestos, for example, might serve to initiate the formation of cancer cells in the lungs, but because of effective immune system responses, metastasis is held in check. Unfortunately, habits such as smoking undermine this immune system response, as the carcinogens in the cigarette smoke contribute to and accelerate the derangement of lung tissue. It is thus no surprise to find that in the U.S. one third of all cancer deaths per annum are directly linked to tobacco use. [90]

How exercise can help prevent cancer

In addition to assisting in the prevention of heart attack, exercise and diet have now been shown to assist the body's fight against cancer. One reason why this is so that being overweight and unfit are risk factors associated with lowered immunity and impaired biochemical function. Let us first consider the role of exercise in the prevention of cancer.

In 1985 the American Cancer Society published an informative booklet titled *Taking Control,* in which exercise was explicitly recommended as a protective measure against cancer. More recent research on the topic confirms this recommendation and shows that exercise may serve to reduce the risk of getting cancer in several ways. Although obesity clearly increases the incidence of cancer of the uterus, breast, gall bladder, and colon, the association of ovarian, breast, and endometrial (mucous lining membrane of the uterus) cancers with high levels of dietary fat is now believed to involve hormonal factors of particular relevance to women. The idea is that increases in the intake level of dietary fat are paralleled by increases in the production of the female hormone estrogen. Roughly put, fatter women tend to have higher estrogen levels than leaner women. The problem is that excessive production of estrogen has been shown to cause cancer-disposing abnormalities in the rates of cellular growth in tissues such as those found in the uterus and breasts. Women undergoing estrogen replacement therapy, for example, exhibit a six-fold increase over the "normal" female population in the incidence of cancer of the endometrium.

Other studies indicate that exercise can significantly reduce estrogen levels. This may explain in part why female athletes display a lower incidence of estrogen-induced cancers than do nonathletic females. In a revealing study by

Dr. Rose Frisch of the Harvard School of Public Health, the incidence of breast cancer was nearly two times greater in nonathletic women than in athletic women. Similarly, the incidence of cancer of the reproductive system was shown to be two-and-a-half times greater in the nonathletes. Frisch is careful to emphasize that *long-term, regular exercise* is the key factor in determining the lower incidence of reproductive cancers in females, *not* the intensive forms of sports training which some women engage in sporadically. [91]

As early as 1984 a correlation between lower rates of cancer of the colon and varying levels of exercise was confirmed by Dr. David Garabrant of the University of Southern California. The more active an individual, the less likely the risk of acquiring cancer of the descending colon. Indeed, the incidence of cancer in the descending colon proved to be three times more prevalent among sedentary individuals than among their physically active counterparts. [92] In a more general study of cancer of the colon Dr. John Vera of the State University of New York at Buffalo reported that individuals who worked at sedentary jobs for more than forty percent of their work years had twice the incidence of cancer of the colon than individuals whose long-term occupations involved regular physical activity. [93]

It is now also well established that constipation is associated with increased risk of cancer of the colon. Several studies have demonstrated that exercise can help relieve constipation and thus indirectly reduce the risk of cancer of the colon. Exercise promotes regular and more frequent bowel movements by stimulating the peristaltic action of the intestines. By speeding up the process whereby fecal matter is passed through the large intestine, the available contact time for any carcinogenic waste material with the colon is minimized.

Diet and cancer prevention

A number of studies have shown that overweight people eat no more food than leaner people. Metabolism partly explains the difference in the way in which food is converted and utilized by our bodies. Overweight people almost invariably have a slower metabolism than do lean ones. It is also the case that the sustenance of muscle requires calorie expenditure even at rest, whereas fat does not. Dieting on its own thus does little to effect permanent weight loss. Exercise coupled with dieting, however, significantly increases the chance of permanent weight loss. One key factor in the marriage of exercise and diet is - as we have earlier seen - that exercise can elevate the metabolism for many hours subsequent to the exercise session, thereby ensuring that dieting is far more effective.

In a longitudinal study from 1959-1972 undertaken by the American Cancer Society it was shown that, of he 750,000 people surveyed, the death rate from cancer was significantly higher for those whose bodyweight was forty percent or more above average. [94, 95] Consistent with the estrogen-excess theory described above, the overweight women displayed higher rates of cancer associated with the reproductive organs. Once again, high dietary fat was nominated as the culprit, but not all fats are equally to blame.

Fats in our food come in solid and in liquid form, and these forms are divided into saturated and unsaturated fats. Analysis of fat reveals, however, that there is no fat which is 100% saturated or 100% unsaturated - all fats are combinations of saturated and unsaturated fatty acids. The extent to which a fat is saturated refers to the number of hydrogen atoms which attach to the fatty acids. A fat is called saturated when its fatty acids carry the maximum number of hydrogen atoms. Saturated fats, two examples of which are butter and lard, usually take the form of solids at room temperature. Saturated fats contain large quantities of low-density lipoprotein, a type of cholesterol notorious for clogging the arterial system with deposits, thereby increasing the risk of heart attack. Unsaturated fats have some hydrogen atoms missing and are further classified as monounsaturated (missing one hydrogen atom) and polyunsaturated (missing more than one hydrogen atom). Olive, peanut, and avocado oils are regarded as monounsaturated, while corn, sunflower, and safflower oils are primarily polyunsaturated.

The health trend in recent years has been to avoid saturated fats whenever possible, substituting in their place polyunsaturates such as margarine. The shift from saturated to polyunsaturated fats may have served to reduce the risk of heart disease, but ironically, it may have inadvertently served to increase the risk of cancer. It turns out that when exposed to oxygen, polyunsaturated fats are especially prone to going rancid. This process of deterioration is called "peroxidation," one by-product of which is the formation of chemical substances called "free radicals." Free radicals, however, are toxic metabolic substances which attack cellular membranes, causing cell-structure abnormalities associated with the initiation stage of cancer.

To some extent the human organism is capable of defending itself against the intrusion of free radicals and its defense can be mounted by way of two mechanisms. First, the body can itself produce natural antioxidants such as superoxide dismutase which tend to counter the deleterious activity of free radicals. The second mode of defense - more controversial than the first - is the consumption of dietary antioxidants which attach themselves to free radicals, thereby impeding their attacks on cellular membranes. Among nutrients presumed to act as antioxidant agents are vitamins A, B-complex, C, E, beta carotene, and the minerals manganese, zinc, and selenium

Consumed in moderate quantities, it would seem that monounsaturates provide one of the best sources of dietary fat. The reason for this is that they do not generate the problem of "free radicals" associated with polyunsaturates on the one hand and they do not contain the low-density lipoproteins associated with hardening of the arteries on the other. On the contrary, they contain *high density lipoprotein* which (as is now well established) actually assists in lowering the level of low density lipoprotein.

What you can do to prevent cancer

It is becoming increasingly apparent that cancer is a disease of modern civilization. Our contemporary lifestyle and the environmental factors to which it has given birth have worked conjointly to disrupt normal cellular function on the one hand, while suppressing the immune system on the other. The combination is—as the cancer epidemic betrays—utterly catastrophic.

We are not helpless in the face of this challenge, despite the massive environmental reformation which must accompany the changes we make to our own lifestyle. No one is responsible for everything, but everyone is responsible for something.

In the light of current research and the foregoing discussion the following recommendations represent a useful set of cancer-prevention guidelines.

1. Exercise is a crucial and much-neglected factor in the prevention of cancer. The key here is long-term, regular exercise, capable of strengthening the muscles of the body on the one hand, while improving cardiovascular fitness on the other. A systematic program of circuit weight training undertaken four to five days per week can be particularly valuable. Such a program will be effective on its own but can be coupled with aerobic movements to reduce elevated bodyfat and estrogen levels further.

2. Excessive bodyfat levels significantly increase the risk of cancer. In addition to regular exercise, low-fat diets assist in the control of bodyfat. It is estimated that approximately forty percent of the nutrients contained in the diet of the average American derive from fats. Australians cannot be far behind. It is important to remember that not all fats are equal. Saturated and polyunsaturated fats have been implicated in the initiation phase of several types of cancer. Monounsaturates offer an alternative. If you find yourself consuming large quantities of polyunsaturated fats, it may be advisable to introduce antioxidant supplements such as Vitamin A / betacarotene into your diet. In any case the total fats consumed should make up no more than twenty percent of your entire diet.

3. Be more aware of the non-fatty foods you consume. Some people fastidiously avoid fatty foods but take little interest in what *remains* of their diet when the fat intake has been reduced. *Total diet awareness is essential in the prevention of cancer.* Consistent with our earlier discussion, some concrete suggestions are appropriate.

a. Be sure to consume plenty of cruciferous vegetables, as they have been shown to contain enzymes capable of preventing colorectal, stomach, and lung cancers. Cruciferous vegetables include cabbage, broccoli, cauliflower, and brussel sprouts.

b. Add sufficient dietary fiber to your diet. Adequate fiber intake assists cancer prevention by diluting the concentration of bile acids in the colon implicated in the formation of colon tumors, and by decreasing intestinal transit time, thereby minimizing the exposure time of the colon to irritants and carcinogens.

c. Get plenty of Vitamin C in your diet, as it is believed to inhibit the formation of nitrosamines, potent carcinogens associated with stomach cancer. Vitamin C food sources include citrus fruits, melons, and currants. 'Red' fruits such as strawberries, watermelon, and pink grapefruit are not only rich in Vitamin C but contain a red pigment called lycopene. Although nutritionally inert, lycopene has been shown to function (not unlike beta-carotene) as an antioxidant, capable of reversing early changes in epithelial tissue associated with the initiation stage of cancer.

4. Give up smoking. In addition to carcinogens cigarettes contain over six thousand toxic chemicals. Damage to and constriction of the blood vessels is caused by the nicotine in cigarette smoke, while the carbon monoxide in the smoke

decreases the capacity of the body to deliver oxygen to the cells, thereby causing premature fatigue and possible suppression of those immune functions which depend on sufficient oxygen supply. When you go to light up your next cigarette, you may find your habit easier to resist knowing that 83% of all lung cancers and 30% of all other types of cancer are associated with smoking. Don't let your health go up in smoke.

Exercise highs

It has been shown that exercise can also contribute to our mental well-being. Although the physiological connections between exercise and depression are not entirely clear, a considerable literature has accumulated on the benefits of exercise for stress management and associate forms of depression. Dr. Rod Dishman of the University of California reports one recent Norwegian study, for example, in which a group of patients suffering from clinical depression responded more positively to psychotherapy when it was accompanied with regular exercise sessions. One theory proposes that vigorous exercise increases the amount of noradrenaline - a hormone which is known to affect moods - by four to six times. Coupled with increased levels of endorphin production in the brain during exercise, it is likely that feelings of well-being and mood elevation will be further enhanced. [96, 97]

When all is said, it is clear that sensible exercise should be as much part of our lifestyle as sensible eating. In recognizing the benefits of exercise we may be better placed also to appreciate the benefits of the wholistic lifestyle of which it is meant to be a part. Exercise is not in itself the end of the story, but it can be the beginning of a story which tells of a happier, healthier, and longer life.

Pre-conditions of health: The moral dimensions

To achieve the goal of health for all, we have observed that much needs to be done to heighten public awareness of the extent to which environmental conditions and our lifestyles contribute to the maintenance of health and the prevention of disease. Such improvements, however, will have little effect unless certain basic humanistic requirements are met. The concept of global health cannot be realized in a world where there exist invidious forms of social inequality and injustice, civil and international unrest, where illiteracy exists and where housing is inadequate. Unless these basic human needs can be fulfilled, social growth and development will inevitably be stifled. As Abraham Maslow asserted, "the single wholistic principle that binds together the multiplicity of human motives is the tendency for a new and higher need to emerge as the lower need fulfills itself by being sufficiently gratified." [98] Unless survival needs are met, individuals will have no energy to spare for needs at a higher level such as assuming responsibility for their own health, much less the health of the community. Let us consider briefly these moral dimensions of health promotion.

Equal health opportunity for all

Fundamental to the idea of health for all lies the principle that all beings have an equal right to health. This right is in fact enshrined in the Universal

Declaration of Human Rights (1948), and the World Health Organization has been one of the most active agencies, along with the United Nations Organization, in promoting this right. But how can such an ideal be realized given that there is gross inequality in lifestyles and budgeting for health care throughout the world? Even within a particular country it is not uncommon to see inequality in access to health care facilities. Those who are privately insured or who can afford the costs, for example, have less time to wait for treatment compared with those who can ill afford insurance or the costs of even basic medical care.

The World Health Organization draws attention to the problem of inequalities which arise even in the apparently affluent countries. "Even in the most highly developed countries, 17 years less life expectancy has been found among the lowest social class compared with the highest." [99] Thus a major task in any National health program is to establish a policy for the long-term reduction of any unjustified existing social inequalities if the goal of health for all is to be realized in the next eleven years.

Peace for all

The World Health Organization considers that "war is the most serious of all threats to health". [100] Millions of people have died and are dying today from starvation and a host of other diseases in war-torn countries. In this decade several wars are raging and national tragedies such as the current situations of famine in Ethiopia and Mozambique are accentuated by war. While the wars go on the efforts of aid agencies to distribute food and medicines is hindered, and the chances of establishing education programs to promote health in these areas are almost nonexistent.

Putting actual war aside, the resources of a government that are directed to defense and armaments provide strenuous competition for health resources. In 2003, the United Nations Department of Public information estimated that 60 billion dollars per annum is spent annually to provide safe water for the whole world˙ however, when compared to the United States budget for military affairs alone, is 33 times less in its overall expenditure. Many of the developing countries, particularly those which have gained independence since World War II, are suffering internal wars and political unrest and have a significantly higher military budget than they do a health budget. Banoub has pointed out, that the ratio of health expenditure to military expenditure is about "1:8 in low income countries." [101]

Peace is indeed a complex concept, and its analysis clearly involves more than affirming the absence of war. Peace instills a positive sense of well-being, social confidence, and security in all persons. Today we see health problems related not solely to actual war, but to the threat of war. Such fears have been particularly evident in Europe. The level of anxiety and apprehension over nuclear war in many Europeans has been shown to manifest itself in health breakdown. As Solantus reported, 79 percent of twelve-year-olds listed the threat of nuclear war among their three greatest fears, and 8 percent of their sample of twelve-to eighteen-year-olds mentioned that they thought about the threat of nuclear war "daily." [102]

Banoub has charged that no satisfactory research has been carried out on the morality and morbidity of war. If the health sectors of national governments took upon themselves the task of making objective assessments of these matters, it could well highlight to governments the utter futility of war. Moreover, it is hard to see how the health facilities of any country could meet the medical demands associated with war, especially a nuclear war with thousands upon thousands of causalities. Banoub suggests:

> Acute, restorative and rehabilitative surgery for causalities among civilian and armed forces are diverting resources from primary health care and public health services. . . . If data were available on these matters, perhaps they would prove wars and military operations to be the most serious of all epidemics in some regions. [103]

Summary

When all is said, it is clear that contemporary society faces a momentous challenge. The real tasks confronting society are not the cosmetic ones of boiling water or buying aeration devices for our taps, though these may of course be helpful in the short run. The real challenge is to redefine the notions of progress and technological achievement which have left us the legacy of contaminated lakes and streams, skies darkened with pollution, processed foods, too little exercise, social inequality, and social unrest. We need to rethink our values and develop the strength of will required to act on them. Like the giant Antaeus in the Greek legend, we must come to understand that to maintain our true strength and health; we must not lose contact with the earth. We need to recast our vision of knowledge and exchange our insatiable desire to subdue and control nature for a new consciousness in which we join nature in partnership and the stewardship of renewal.

CHAPTER 5

From the individual to the social body: Community as good medicine

Growing dissatisfaction with conventional medicine and health care has led to considerable reflection upon the inadequacy of the bioreductionist approach to medicine. Given the purported role of education in the advancement of world health, it will be instructive to turn our attention now to the emergent concept of primary health care, as it plays a major role in promoting the connection between education and health. In the present chapter we will be concerned to introduce the concept of primary health care, tracing its evolution and projecting its potential development in the context of future health care practices. Within this context the relation between health care and social justice arises, and we will in what follows try to get a clearer idea of what this relation is. The other question which comes into relief in this context pertains to the issue of rights and responsibilities for health. For example, if people are supposed to be responsible for the maintenance and protection of their own health care then to what extent can they legitimately expect the provision of health care by the community in which they live as a *right*?

The emergence of primary health care

By the time of the sixth global health promotion conference in Bangkok in 2005 it was generally recognized by health professionals involved that although conventional medicine has assisted in advancing the health of the population its promise to ameliorate the health problems confronting contemporary society were still to be fulfilled. [1]

The exorbitant sums of money being directed to health care were not - as we saw in chapter 2 - leading to improved health status for the community as a whole. Even if one grants that the wealthy in developed countries enjoy a high standard of health care, it is evident that the majority of the world population remains grossly disadvantaged. On this point March writes:

> Remarkable improvements have been made in health status worldwide over the last century, but these improvements have not been shared equally. The gap between rich and poor nations has widened, as have inequities within countries, between urban and rural, men and women, and young and old. [2]

Having undertaken a careful study of the world health situation, as far back as 1973, the World Health Organization came to the conclusion that many of the health services which should be improving health were not doing so, and that large portions of the global population did not have access to health services, or at best had limited access. In many areas health services were acting in isolation from other community agencies and departments which also contribute to human well-being, such as education, communications, and agriculture. The main reason for this was the reliance of health services on highly technical equipment provided in central locations, thus excluding those in outlying areas from obtaining health care.

It was apparent that the bioreductionist, high-tech approach to health care had not only proven to be medically ineffective but had inadvertently caused an infelicitous disequilibrium in the type and delivery of health services. Thus the infrastructure and availability of health personnel and equipment were most diffuse at the level of interface closest to the community. The net result was a lack of proper balance between promotive, preventive, curative, restorative, and supportive functions of the overall health care services. *Promotive* health services seek to maintain the health of individuals by encouraging a lifestyle which is conducive to health. *Preventive* functions of the health service are involved in such practices as immunization and ensuring sanitary measures adequate to inhibit the development of disease. The *curative* measures are directed towards complete recovery from disease without morbidity. The *restorative* function aims at returning a patient to the same level of health at which he or she functioned prior to a specific illness; for example, a patient with chronic respiratory disease will never be cured, but following an acute episode of pneumonia will be returned to a state of health no worse than that which he or she has experienced in the past. *Supportive* care is extended to those who will have ongoing contact with health services due to chronic illness and is aimed at enabling those persons, and their family and friends to live in a manner which allows them to realize their potential within the limitations of their illness. Such supportive services may also be involved in the care of the dying and be extended to their family and friends. The focus of health care has for the most part, in recent times, concentrated on the curative and restorative functions at the expense of the other equally vital components of health care.

The World Health Organization is not the only body which has expressed concern over the state of the world's health. Groups such as the Non-Aligned Nations, the Organization of African Unity, the European Economic Community, UNICEF, and the World Bank, as well as many national bodies, have expressed dissatisfaction with the status of health worldwide or in respect of their own countries. The common conclusion at which all these organizations arrived, was that a fully functional health service *cannot by provided by the health sector alone,* "but is closely interlinked with all aspects of socioeconomic development." [3] Thus it is only through the coordinated efforts of health and related sectors such as education, coupled with strong political will and community consensus, that the goal of improved health for the general population can be realized. Thus emerges the concept of "primary health care" as central to the enterprise of health.

The 1977 Alma-Ata declaration presented primary health care in the context of social justice, recognizing that the bases of health and disease both rest firmly on the foundations of social, economic, cultural, and political development. By encompassing a more wholistic view of health than the bioreductionist model offers, primary health care takes into account the contributions to global health made by the individual, the family, and the community. The concept of primary health is thus sufficiently comprehensive to view health from a global perspective and not merely from the limited vantage of the health problems confronting developed or undeveloped communities. Indeed, it is a fundamental tenet of primary health that in order to realize the goal of health for all, each nation must identify and plan to overcome its own peculiar set of health problems. In 1985 the World Health Organization affirmed that:

> Primary health care is essential health care made accessible at a cost that the country and the community can afford, with methods that are practical, scientifically sound and socially acceptable. Everyone in the community should have access to it, and everyone should be involved in it. [3]

Questions arise, however, concerning the extent to which methods which are deemed to be "scientifically sound" are consistent with the wholistic emphasis of primary health care. The concept of wholesome in this work encompasses the idea of individuals in constant interaction with their total physical and cultural environment. Science and technology are part of the cultural environment and it is by no means intended that the scientific contribution to health care should be entirely excluded. As will become explicit in chapter 6, part of the goal of education is to enlighten those involved in health care so that they are able to recognize for themselves what scientific methods are appropriate to the particular health goals they seek to realize. The extent to which high-technology medicine is inimical to health depends partly upon the *health needs* of the community on the one hand and the *nature* of the technology on the other. For example, it would be indefensible to provide nuclear medical facilities in an isolated village which does not have clean water and adequate sanitary measures. Indeed, given the *nature* of nuclear medicine, it may be that its use is extremely limited in any situation. Wholistic heal care, as we envisage it, does not condemn unreservedly the use of scientific technology, but rather seeks to place it in a perspective which is appropriate to the health needs of the global community. When this is done, the use of scientific technology becomes what we call "self-limiting." The full analysis of this concept will be given later.

The services and objectives of primary health care go beyond the bioreductionist aims of responding to and curing disease. Primary health care is concerned to emphasize the prevention and promotion of ways in which communities and individuals can take action for themselves to ensure and practice measures which serve to improve health.

In 1980 Fry suggested that primary health care was actually an "old-new" branch of health care. He went so far as to opine that while the concept of primary care had long been around, it has become fashionable to talk about it only since the World Health Organization gave it its strong endorsement at the Alma-Ata conference. Referring to primary health care Fry has written:

> It has been the Cinderella of medicine waiting for a Prince Charming to rediscover it and give it its rightful place in the professional hierarchy, Lo and behold! in September 1978 there was a great ball at Alma-Ata . . . and the World Health Organization was the unlikely Prince Charming. [4]

It has been further suggested by Fry that the idea of primary health care has been resurrected in the hope that it will provide services available to the public at less expense than hospital services. Notwithstanding Fry's point about the antiquity of the concept of primary care, what seems to be new is the notion that primary health care can provide the organizing framework for the development of a global health system. On this view health is to be regarded as a dynamic process of interaction with the natural and social environment expressed in different ways by different persons throughout the entire world. As Litsios puts it:

> What is new is the recognition that primary health care must be the central focus of the total health system that takes the meaning of health in its widest sense. [5]

What issues does primary health care address?

Consistent with a wholistic and more comprehensive approach to health, the issues addressed by primary health care are similarly broad in nature. The main issues are those related to the problems of providing the five functional components of health care alluded to previously: promotion, prevention, cure, restoration, and support. Such services will, by their very nature, vary from country to country, as they must reflect and be conditioned by the economic and cultural values of each country. It may even be the case that within a country the orientation of health services will vary somewhat as they reflect the differing social values and economic standards of various segments of the community. In addition to this, primary health care comprises the following services: provision of maternal and child care, family planning, immunization against infectious disease, control of local endemic diseases, and education about prevention and control of diseases, coupled with the promotion and reflective interpretation of health lifestyles. Primary health care will also address itself to the issue of providing treatment for common diseases and injuries, as well as being involved in the restorative and supportive aspects of care required by the members of the specific community.

Primary health care is regarded as the first point of contact that an individual or community has with a health care facility. It does, however, have several other important dimensions. Firstly, there is the notion of continuing care. Implicit in this is the idea of responsibility shared with the individual or community over many years, and this suggests the idea of defined geographical areas of practice. The interests of primary health care are also of a more comprehensive nature than conventional medical care, which is primarily directed to intervention following the onset of disease. In primary health care, that care is directed to the physical, psychological, spiritual, and social needs of the individual or community *whether or not disease* in the conventional sense is present. The role of primary health in this sense is somewhat reminiscent, as Fry would suggest, of the involvement in the community of the local general practitioner prior to the age of specialization. [7] This specialization, however, brought with it the process of increasing depersonalization to which we referred earlier. People came to be viewed as receptacles for the specific disease, with which they were afflicted, and a person was reduced to a diagnostic category - a reduction deliberately avoided in the wholistic orientation to primary health care.

Primary health care is not an institutional leg of crisis medicine; it is not in this regard intended to provide facilities for anything other than treatment of minor illnesses or accidents. Those diseases or injuries of crisis requiring more substantial intervention would be referred to a *secondary* level of care, where basic diagnostic, surgical, and pharmaceutical services are provided. In turn, *tertiary* health care facilities are those which provide for advanced technological diagnostic interventionist measures and serve to receive people referred from primary or secondary care facilities as the need arises. When appropriate, these people would be returned to the local primary health care facility for long-term care, cooperative between the individual and the health care system as a functional whole. The point here is that the contribution to overall health made by conventional medicine would be minimized, and the nature of its intervention reviewed to coordinate with the approach of primary care, not the other way around.

One of the essential features of primary health care is clearly the involvement of the community, both as individuals and a collective group. To be successful, primary health care relies on the community for resources and support. The measure of community support is seen as a measure of community commitment to the goal of improving overall health. The term *involvement* is used in preference to *participation* because it implies a deeper and more personal commitment to the idea of health by the members of a community. Through involvement individuals and families assume more responsibility for their community's health and are able to contribute in a meaningful way to the development of their culture.

In 1977 Rogers outlined eight basic capabilities which must be exhibited by primary health care if this service is to be adequately delivered on a national level [8], standards that contain to apply within the context of primary health, in the twenty first century. In his original work Rogers concentrated on the specific role of the physician in primary health care, though his ideas can be extended to include those which are more compatible with a notion of wholism in health.

1. There should be ready access to the primary health care facility, whether staffed by professional or nonprofessional health workers. Accessibility implies the continuing and organized supply of care that is geographically, financially, culturally, and functionally within easy reach of the whole community.
2. The facility should have the resources to identify potentially serious problems and be able to provide properly for them, possibly by referral to a secondary or tertiary level of care, as well as to meet the daily requirements of

the area and its inhabitants. This involves having health worker trained to recognize the signs and symptoms of common or uncomplicated diseases and simple injuries. The same individual should be able to treat these basic infirmities, or, if unable to do so, to recognize the need for referral and to take the appropriate action. Additionally, this implies having at hand the basic equipment necessary to diagnose and treat such conditions as outlined, and access should be available to appropriate means of communication for referral as needed.

3. The facility should provide soundly based support for those whom it serves, including the provision of medical knowledge and technology, where appropriate.
4. Care should be provided on a continuing or long-term basis.
5. The distribution of care should be on a reasonably equitable basis. That is, health care should be distributed so as to achieve a reduction in the gap between those who have ready access to health care and those who do not, in order that an acceptable level of health may be attained by all.
6. The delivery system must be stable and self-renewing. Those who work in it should be willing to stay, and there must be incentive for others to enter.
7. It must be compatible with the life, culture, and needs of the people with whom it shares the responsibility for health. The delivery system should be able to adapt to various health concerns as they arise in different locals and regions. Rural concerns may well be different from urban concerns, for example, and the health problems of developing regions will, as we have seen, be different from those of developed ones.

It must be able to compete for resources with other social needs and to cooperate with the bodies involved in the sharing of those resources to the best advantage of the community as a whole.

A similar list of eight conditions thought to constitute good primary health care is put forward by Fry. For Fry primary health can be described by a series of A's which ensure that it is:

Available
Accessible
Approachable
Acceptable
Affordable
Applicable
Attainable
Assessable [9]

In essence, then, primary health care must be *present* in a community. It has also to be of such a nature that it is *understood* by and is *relevant* to the needs of the local community, which in turn must be able to *afford* the facilities which primary health care seeks to provide. Moreover, primary health care must be structured in such a way that it admits of *evaluation* on an ongoing basis. Open to the public scrutiny, its deficiencies may be recognized and corrected, and its strengths may continue to be fostered. Clearly, primary health care involves considerably more than the basic health services to which most people in developed countries have access. Given that few people can avail themselves even of basic health services in developing countries, the introduction of primary health care would go a long way towards advancing the general level of health in such countries.

How do primary health care and basic health services differ?

Basic health services, with which most people are familiar, consist of a network of institutions run by the government as part of a country's administrative system. Basic health services provide certain indispensable medical treatment and preventive services to individuals. Such services are rendered by professional and nonprofessional staff who have been selected without consultation with the community they serve, and the community is not usually involved in the decisions and actions taken to improve its health. Services such as these usually begin at a central point and radiate to the periphery; that is, they are usually based at a high-technology hospital and do not take into account the resource limitations of the peripheral community which they are attempting to serve.

The World Health organization considers that basic health services "do not necessarily attempt to identify and use appropriate technology." [10] "Appropriate" technology means techniques and equipment that are adapted to local needs and acceptable to those who use them and those for whom they are used. Further, for technology to be appropriate it must be able to be utilized and maintained within the resources of the community in which it is used.

Basic health services do not take account of the socioeconomics aspects of health, nor is it customary for them to have sufficient regard for the activities in which the health sector and other relevant sectors could collaborate for the achievement of a common goal. As the World health Organization has stressed:

> Health development and socioeconomic development are inseparably linked, progress in health leading to and at the same time depending on socioeconomic progress. Health development implies coordination at all levels between activities in the health sector and activities in other social an economic sectors such as education, agriculture, industry, housing, public works, water supply, and communications. Hence the need for intersectorial action. [11]

Primary health care, on the other hand, takes into account all the foregoing issues, and has its goals set for it by the community which it is intended to serve. The challenge of primary health care for the community is the placing of the responsibility for self-care on each member of that community. This implies that largely unorganized health activities and health-related decision making will be carried out by individuals, families, friends, and work associates. Such decisions include the maintenance of health, prevention of disease, self-diagnosis, and treatment, including medication and follow-up care after contact with the health services at any level. Such a weighty responsibility cannot be taken without thoughtful and informed preparation by those involved, and such preparation requires what might be called "education for health."

The several dimensions of primary health care can best be summarized by drawing on the words of the World Health Organization.

> Primary health care is the key to achieving an acceptable level of health throughout the world in the foreseeable future as part of social development and in the spirit of social justice. It is equally valid for all countries, from the most to the least developed, though the form it takes will vary according to the political, economic, social and cultural patterns. [12]

While primary health care is equally valid for developing and developed countries, there are differences to be faced by these two types of nations. One urgent problem which is common to both is how best to utilize the resources which are made available for health care. Emphasizing the similarities and the differences, Fry writes:

> In developing countries there are shortages of all resources and those medical and health resource that are available often are misused and wasted. In developed countries there may be too many medical and health resources which often are misused and wasted. [13]

Fry's point is further stressed by the United States Institute of Medicine in 2008 who stated that "30 to 40 cents of every dollar spent on health care is for costs associated with overuse, underuse, misuse, duplication, system failures, unnecessary repetition, poor communication and inefficiency."[14]

Health: A human right or an individual responsibility?

Implicit in the foregoing discussion of primary health care is a philosophical premise which should now be made explicit. One important component in the philosophical foundations of primary health care relates to its justification by appeal to the concept of social justice and rights theory. While acknowledging that the problem or the whole host of problems concerning rights and duties impinges upon a complex domain of philosophical scholarship whose elaboration is beyond the scope of this work, we are convinced that a brief discussion of the issues in regard to the "right to health" will confirm the philosophical impetus to primary health care. The basic issue arises in considering the extent to which individuals can expect health care as a *right,* given - on the view of primary health care we have proposed - that they are *responsible* for the maintenance and protection of their own health. The other questions whether victims of disease can, in some moral sense or other, be blamed for their failure of health thus becomes particularly pertinent. When all is said, the problem or host of problems in respect of the right to health, the responsibility for health, and the moral culpability attached to its failure figure prominently in the elucidation of the philosophical foundations of health education. If one accepts that people are responsible for their own health, then one must also accept that there is a responsibility on the part of the community to ensure that individuals make educationally informed decisions about issues relating to their health, whether in the workplace, the home, or in he wider physical and cultural environment. Similarly, if health is a responsibility shared between the individual and the wider society (e.g., the government and health care professionals), then education becomes of paramount importance in ensuring that each individual is prepared to contribute not only to the maintenance of his or her own health but to the communal dialogue which will shape the health policies and condition the interventionist practices of the professionals.

The concept of social justice and health

Justice is a complex concept and one usually associated with law and lawfulness; yet it has a broader sense closer to the notion of fairness. As Stanley Benn indicates, "justice presupposes people pressing claims and justifying them by rules or standards." [15] On Benn's view, the amenability of justice to justification distinguishes it from *charity*, *benevolence,* and *generosity*; justice excludes people from claiming alms or gifts as a *right.* Let us examine the concept of justice more closely as it relates to primary health care.

One of the more influential concepts of justice has been developed by John Rawls, who defined justice in terms of "the role of principles in assigning rights and social duties and in defining the appropriate division of social advantages." [16] Rawls's theory of justice provides a comprehensive discussion of rights and duties and has thus been adopted by a number of health professionals as the accepted rationale for the distribution of health resources and the rights of access to it. [17]

Rawls develops a carefully articulated set of moral principles in regard to which it is presumed that free and equal persons, with no self-interest other than a rational expectation of enhancing their own life prospects, would be likely to accept as fundamental terms for their mutual societal regulation. His theory assumes also that the individuals involved are not biased by prior knowledge of how the social accident of their birth will affect the outcome of their choice. In this sense, his theory of social justice is closely connected with the theory of rational choice. Rawls acknowledges the unpredictability of individual circumstances, and he makes a clear distinction between *inequality* and *injustice.* He states that the distribution of "primary social goods" may be unequal and still be just if these inequalities somehow work to everyone's more general advantage. This last point betrays his disposition to utilitarianism, and inclination concerning which he has been criticized by several detractors.[18]

The major principles of justice, according to Rawls, are, first, that every person has a right to the maximum degree of personal and political liberty; and second, that the social and economic inequalities are *just* if everyone has an equal opportunity for social achievement, and if disproportionate socioeconomic gains by the most advantaged in society also help to improve the situation of the least advantaged. Rawls does not give a great deal of specific consideration to health issues, but in his passing comments, he does refer to health status as a condition not primarily controlled by social order, although affected by it. In other words, the health status of the members of a given society cannot be predetermined and maintained by social order, but rather the level of health will be affected by the provision, or lack of provision regarding health and health care within that social order.

John Bryant, Former Deputy Assistant Secretary for International Health, has written extensively on health education and social justice. He regards health education as one of the basic requirements of the adequate provision of health services, and any statements he makes in relation to health care should be taken to include health education. Bryant rests his argument for distribution of health care on Rawlsian foundations for the theory of justice. Consider Rawl's claim that "all social primary goods - liberty and opportunity, income and wealth, and the bases of self-respect - are to be distributed equally unless an unequal distribution of any or all of these goods is to the advantage of the least favored." [19] Bryant translates this general principal of justice into words specifically applicable to health care thus: "whatever health services are available should be equally available to all unless unequal distribution would be to the advantage to the least favored." [20]

Stewart objects, however, that Bryant is incorrect in construing Rawl's theory in such a manner, for on this interpretation of health care services, it would follow that the sickest would receive the most care. [21] Stewart asserts that Bryant's interpretation is misleading on three counts. First, Rawls never mentions receipt of optimal level of health services as an aspect of equal right to personal liberty. Second, Rawls clearly indicates that degrees of health, like levels of intelligence, are primarily a property of nature and not an endemic feature of the social order. Third, Rawls is primarily concerned to extend the concept of justice to those circumstances which allow the accrual of benefits to those already more advantaged because, in so doing, it also benefits the less advantaged. Stewart argues that if Bryant's use of Rawls's theory in this manner is taken into its logical conclusion, then health resources would be entirely used for treating the sickest among the population to the exclusion of prevention and research. In a subsequent paper Bryant explicitly denies this, asserting that in his original paper, he had in fact pointed to these three aspects of health care as being essential constituents of a primary health care program across all levels of community, including those programs with a dearth of health resources to those with a relative oversupply of resources. [22]

It is no part of our purpose to assess the exegetical accuracy of either Bryant's or Stewart's interpretations of Rawls. We would in any case suggest that the debate has been proscribed prematurely. To focus on such a narrow aspect of Rawls's theory is in itself myopic, as is the attempt to base the rationale for distribution of health care on a global scale on this one Rawlsian principle alone. Our suggestion is that the discussion be extended to include such questions as:

1. Is the misdistribution of health services on a global scale an acceptable social phenomenon?
2. What are the consequences in the long and short term of such misdistribution of these resources?

3. Is it applicable to consider the distribution of health resources on a global scale in light of a philosophy of justice that is steeped in European tradition?

These and many other questions could and should be raised in reference in distributive justice and health care. If the problem of adequate distribution of health care resources is to be resolved on a worldwide scale in a satisfactory manner for all peoples of all cultures, we will need a more comprehensive theory of distribution than that offered by Bryant. As Benn indicated, justice in distribution is not based on a claim as a right but on a claim justified by a rule or a standard. For example, he notes that "no one can claim alms or gifts as a right." [23] We are thus brought full circle to the consideration of health and health care as a right to be claimed by individuals or as a joint responsibility to be shared with the wider social order.

Right versus responsibility

Many writers, both from Eastern and Western cultures, have expressed the idea of reciprocal responsibility when discussing human rights. Spengler, for example regarded every genuine right as a product of duty. [24] Rawls himself makes frequent mention of the notion of autonomy being reciprocal with responsibility, particularly in relation to the Law, and this principle could equally be extended to health. He states, "everyone is autonomous yet responsible."

In a letter to Sir Julian Huxley, then Director General of UNESCO, M. K. Gandhi wrote: "I learnt from my illiterate but wise mother that all rights to be deserved and preserved come from duty well done." Also from a Hindu perspective, a similar sentiment is expressed by Puntambekar who believes that human freedom requires as its counterpart human virtue and control. Chung-Shu Lo, in writing on human rights from a Chinese perspective, expressed a like notion when he wrote "that each by making the most of himself can at the same time contribute best to the world at large." [24] From even these few selected writings, it is clear that the notion of "rights reciprocated by responsibility" emerges independently of its philosophical justification as an idea entrenched cross-culturally. Appreciation of this point reinforces Benn's claim that just distribution is based on claims supported by rules or standards rather than claims based on rights alone.

The notion that health care is a *right* has been bandied about at least since the 1930s. In 1948 with the creation of the *Universal Declaration of Human Rights,* at least for member nations of the United Nations Organization, the right to health via an adequate standard of living, and to medical care, was expressed in written terms thus:

> ARTICLE 25. Everyone has the right to a standard of living adequate for health and well-being of himself and his family, including food, clothing, housing and medical care and necessary social services, and the right to security in the event of unemployment, sickness, disability, widowhood, old age or lack of livelihood in circumstances beyond his control.

> (2) Motherhood and childhood are entitled to special care and assistance. All children born in or out of wedlock, shall enjoy the same protection.

Nonetheless, the right to health is a curious and somewhat obscure idea. It quantifies health and suggests that health can be distributed by society to its members on request rather like medicine from a bottle. Reminding us that health cannot be measured out in this way. Colman writes:

> positive health is not something that one human can hand to or require of another. Positive health can be achieved only through intelligent effort. Absent that effort, health professionals can only insulate the individual from more catastrophic results of his ignorance, self-indulgence, or lack of motivation. [26]

Colman is intimating that health can only result from individual willingness to adopt appropriate lifestyles and to put considerable effort into maintaining healthy behavior. Without such effort health professionals can only apply interventionist techniques to limit the consequences of unhealthy behavior.

Fuchs sees the right to *medical care* as more plausible than the notion of the right to *health* as such. [27] He relates medical care to health in the way that schooling is related to wisdom. This recognizes that no society can make everybody wise but that every society has the potential, if it has the political will, to make education and schooling freely available. In the same way no government, now or in the foreseeable future, can make all its citizens healthy, but can, with political will and effort, make available health care services at a cost which is affordable and in a manner which is acceptable to all its citizens.

The right to *health care* is itself also a curious idea. The historical concept of individual rights conveys the implication that governments or other authorities have a clear duty to refrain from interfering with individual liberty. The concept of the right to health care takes a decidedly different tack - it implies that someone has a positive duty, derived from an unwritten social contract, to provide explicit services to the holder of such a right. As Duval points out, medical care is only one small part of the maintenance of health. [28] The concept of primary health care, it will be recalled, implies aspects of care related to promotion, prevention, cure, restoration, and support. Medical care is usually concerned with the curative and restorative aspects of care, but if, as the Declaration of Human Rights asserts, people have a right to medical care and a standard of living that is adequate for health, then equally they have a right to the components of health care that will ensure these rights. If the basic premise is correct that someone or some community has a duty to provide explicit health services to the claimant of the right to health, and given that education for health is endorsed as a vital component of primary health care, then there is clearly a duty on the part of the provider to ensure that education for health is available just as medical care is provided.

Fuchs raises the question, "if people have a *right* to care, do they also have an *obligation* to use it? " [29] He cautions that attempts to raise health levels must not impinge on peoples' rights to be left alone, for even if strict control over health issues does lead to increased life-expectancy, if that life is spent in a "zoo", no matter how well run, it may not be worth living. Fuchs goes on to quote from Rabbi Hillel, who said: "If I am not for myself, who will be for me, but if I am for myself alone, what am I?" [30] Such a statement suggests that all individuals have a responsibility for their own health and also for that of their fellows, and, moreover, a responsibility to ensure that the environment in which they live is as conductive to health as possible.

The general attitude to health is well expressed in the words of a popular song of the sixties written by Joni Mitchell, "You don't know what you've got 'til it's gone." Most people do not worry about their health until they lose it. Some of the reasons why people disregard their health include the denial of death and disease, and the hedonism of instant gratification of day-to-day life. In addition to this is the feeling perpetuated in modern Western society that the advances of science and technology will be able to correct any health problems that may arise. There is also a prevailing attitude that to live into old age is not desirable if that life is to be spent in misery as the body and mind slowly degenerate. So the ethos of "eat, drink and be merry, for tomorrow we may die" has come to permeate the philosophy by which many still live.

In 1977 Knowles reinforced the basic thrust of these ideas by exposing the apparent disinterest of some physicians in promoting a positive attitude to health by their own bad example. [31] The one person to whom most people go if they are ill or need advice is often a walking health hazard. Physicians have also - as we have seen - concentrated on curative measures rather than on the wholistic aspects of health care. It would be misguided to apportion to them blame for their commitment to bioreductionism given that medical education has traditionally been reductionist. The technological fallacy or the pervasive view that a scientific high-technology solution can be found for all problems, including technological ones, still holds many a medical mind captive. As Ivan Illich noted: "the professional practice or physicians cannot be credited with the elimination of old forms of mortality, nor ought it to be blamed for the increased expectancy of life spent suffering from new diseases." [32]

Indeed the responsibility for the propagation of high-tech medicine often lies with the patients themselves, who attend the doctor and demand medication or some technologically invasive investigation for their condition and who, if this is not forthcoming, deride the doctor as incompetent. People come - as we have seen - to regard their bodies rather like their motor cars or their washing machines, which can be poorly cared for, then taken to the repair man and mended. Just as many people surrender the responsibility for the maintenance of their cars to the mechanic, so too, they surrender the maintenance of their bodies to the doctor, just as they often yield up the responsibility for their minds to the psychiatrist.

Illich argues that people have been denied the right to accept the responsibility for their own health as this pervasive attitude toward science and technology has increasingly dominated medicine. As we observed in the previous chapter, highly technological medical care has removed from people their autonomous ability to cope with nature and created in its place a dependence on the institutional practice of invasive and often destructive medicine. As Illich stated:

> "this dependence on professional intervention tends to impoverish the non-medical health supporting and healing aspects of the social and physical environments, and tends to decrease the organic and psychological coping ability of ordinary people." [33]

If "recuperation of personal responsibility for health care were made the major goal of legislation," the debate regarding health care could be salvaged. [34] Like Knowles, and Colman, Illich regards the attainment and maintenance of health as a task requiring effort for which each individual is ultimately responsible. Knowles indicated that one person's freedom in health matters is another's shackle in taxes and insurance premiums. The Better Health Commission in Australia (1986) echoed this sentiment when it said: "One person's right to indulge in self-destructive behavior - say, smoking - can become another's shackle in the form of higher premiums or taxes."[35] Thus the right to health care becomes a justified claim only if all individuals also accept the responsibility for maintenance of their own health. This does not mean that people will have to shoulder this burden alone, but that they must be willing to see and to accept that they must share equally with others the responsibility of health care.

Success in the task of attaining and maintaining health comes as a result of self-awareness, self-discipline, and inner resources by which each person regulates his or her daily rhythms, actions, diet, and reproduction. The knowledge to do this, Illich claims, comes from peers and elders, and in a world of optimal health people do not require bureaucratic interference to mate, give birth, live, or die. However, if people have become so dependent on the present practice of high-technology medicine and so far removed from accepting the responsibility for their own lives, as Illich suggests, then it is entirely possible that peers and elders are no longer in a position to pass on the knowledge required for healthy living and rational decision-making in matters of health. The peers and elders of the present are also steeped in the belief that the only valid claims to knowledge are those based - as we have observed earlier - on the bioreductionist approach to medicine - and as such, will perpetuate in their teachings the reliance on methods and practices which presuppose similar scientific claims. Thus their teachings will further encourage the dependence on curative and restorative medicine as practiced widely in the twentieth century, rather than encouraging their "pupils" to accept and utilize their own abilities to cope with the daily happenings of life in general and health in particular.

If it is the case that people are not in a position to pass on the knowledge required for the active participation of individuals in their own health maintenance, then it will require some degree of institutional intervention to encourage the acceptance of this responsibility. The knowledge required to allow the development of self-awareness, self-discipline, and inner resources in individuals must, then, come from those who have recognized the dominance of the scientific worldview and the dependence on technologized medicine in the twentieth century, and who are prepared to cooperate with and not dictate to the community on matters related to health. Such education for health will need to be conceptualized in a different manner from the health education which has taken place in the past. This reconceptualization is a matter to which we will address ourselves in the following chapters of the present work.

Knowles believes that the next major advance in health will be determined by what individuals will be prepared to do for themselves and for society at large. He does, however, believe that individuals have a *right* to expect help with information, access to health services, and minimal financial barriers to health care, thus acknowledging the right of access to health education. The responsibility of the individual should be extended to incorporate such issues as supporting health education programs in schools which stress measures that individuals can take to assume more responsibility for their own health. Furthermore Knowles feels that individuals should agitate to ensure that more of the health budgets of countries be spent on researching health education, its cost and its effectiveness, and ways to make health education less of an *invasion* into the lives of people, becoming rather a fundamental *part* of daily life, as, indeed, is the process of health itself. Knowles acknowledges that health for all is only one goal in the wider social context of life and that other injustices must be addressed in conjunction with the right to health care. Thus education should not only be about matters of health but be extended to the wider social issues arising in people's day-to-day lives. Individuals, Knowles states, should become "knowledgeable enough to participate in public debate" regarding not only health-related concerns, but social issues in general.[36]

If the maintenance of health is an individual responsibility, albeit one shared with the wider society, what are individuals expected to do, in order to maintain their health? It was to this question that Marjorie Keller addressed her article on health and its definition. [37] Keller considered three of what she regarded to be the most comprehensive definitions of health, considering what was required of individuals to meet this weighty obligation. A comprehensive definition for Keller is one which included individual, family, and social aspects, recognized physical, mental, and spiritual well-being, and incorporated consideration of the environment. Drawing heavily on the work of Hanlon, Miller, and Schlosser for her comprehensive definition, she set out the expectations which each author would associate with the achievement of health. She says:

> Hanlon would expect the individual to maintain a state of total physiological and psychological functions within the environment and be able to cope with a variety of internal and external forces, mostly those outside the individual's control.
>
> Miller would expect the individual to achieve special interdependent, harmonic relationships of the physical, mental and spiritual aspects of health that is intertwined with every other individual and society.
>
> Schlosser would expect the individual to develop a meaning in life that includes the realms of physical, mental, aesthetic, interpersonal, social, and spiritual. It

> should be interwoven with love, creativity and self-fulfillment, free from disease and fear of death and dying. [38]

These requirements represent a considerable effort for most people, and one which no doubt will find many falling short. Those who *do* fall short may find themselves being blamed for lacking the qualities which are demanded of them to take responsibility for their own health. It is from this idea of the right to health care carrying with it reciprocal responsibility which has also given rise to the notion of "blaming the victim."

Blaming the victim

According to Crawford the practice of "victim-blaming" reflects a middle-class attitude, perpetuates class structure, and reinforces the political decisions made about the provision and distribution of health care. [39] This practice, which usually accompanies the argument that the individual is responsible for his or her health, implies that "non-persons," the government and industrial corporations, are not responsible for health issues. As Wikler asserts, "The argument for assigning responsibility for health to the individual is often an attempt to absolve these larger institutions of blame for having caused sickness or for having failed to provide care, respectively." [40]

"Victim-blaming" parallels the "limits to medicine" argument put forward by such writers as Illich, McKeown, and Fuchs. Inherent in this claim is the idea that if people lead a healthy lifestyle, eat the right food, exercise, rest, work, and reproduce in appropriate proportions they will be well; if they do not and are unwell, it is their own fault.

The tendency to victim-blaming arises from three factors, according to Crawford. First is the high cost of medical treatment, which has little effect on altering the health status of the world in general. Second, he considers that social production of disease has been politicized, and that industrial pollution which causes many illnesses is accepted because industrial growth is essential to the development of the nation. Crawford is referring here specifically to the United States, but the ideas could well be extended to many other nations preoccupied with industrialization. Third, the fact that health care is regarded as a *right* is a contributing factor to the perpetuation of the practice of victim-blaming. The notion of reciprocal responsibility to protect and promote one's own health is seen as a prerequisite to making a claim to the right to health care. The practice of victim-blaming thus derives from the social obligations affirming rights and responsibilities in respect of them.

Crawford claims that these three factors led to the *ideology* of blaming the victim and suggests that the trend to thrust responsibility onto the individual is concealing the nature of the real causes underlying the current situation in health care.

> But now the cost of individual irresponsibility in health has become prohibitive. The choice is in fact, over the long range, individual responsibility or social failure. [41]

> For once we cannot blame the environment as much as we have to blame ourselves. The problem now is the inability of man to take care of himself. [42]

> We must stop throwing an array of technological processes and systems at lifestyle problems and stop equating more health services with better. . . . People must have the capability and the will to take greater responsibility for their own health. [43]

Crawford intends that these statements should be interpreted by reference to the underlying ideology of victim-blaming, thereby acknowledging that it serves to reinforce political objectives, even though the observations cited may not have been intended for that purpose. Victim-blaming ignores what is known about human behavior and minimizes the importance of the institutional-social-structural assault on health. This ideology convinces people that they should take responsibility for their own health at a time when they are in fact becoming less capable of controlling their own environment. [44]

Blaming the individual in stead of the economic system also reinforces the class structure of work. The failure to maintain health in the workplace is attributed to a personal flaw in the worker: failure to take sufficient precautions or laziness about using protective devices provided, or in some cases the worker's genetic susceptibility to disease are blamed. Often the worker is labeled as "stressed," "overworked" or some such similar tag, and then relaxation training, counseling, or psychological support is offered; but the causes in the work environment go unaltered. Practices which strengthen the ideology of blaming the victim also serve to reduce the compensation payment to the worker who suffers ill health due to the industrial environment or workplace accident.

Victim-blaming is reflected in the lay perceptions of health. In more recent work Crawford, when discussing "health as self-control" points out that health is discussed in terms of self-control and related concepts such as "self-denial," "self-discipline," and "willpower".[45] Similar concepts were discussed by respondents in an interview on perceptions of health and lifestyle change in an Australian survey. [46] Many members of the general public regarded themselves as responsible for their health and blamed themselves for any shortcomings, mostly attributing them to a lack of willpower or self-discipline. As Crawford suggests, these self-blame themes reflect the "general moralization of health under the rubric of self-responsibility." [47] These notions of self-control are deeply embedded in the social structure of most industrialized societies.

Equally embedded in the social structure is the notion of "health-as-release" or freedom from self-control, with many offering ideas that worrying about health and controlling diet, exercise, and other behaviors results in stress which may be equally bad for health. [48, 49] Crawford suggests, and it is difficult to disagree, that modern industrial societies are both the objects and the subjects of two opposing mandates - discipline and pleasure. [50] The overwhelming encouragement to indulge in food, drink, and nicotine are countered by the moral imperative to control these desires. Each individual body has become a battleground between these mandates, each reflecting the social battle for domination. It is not, says Crawford, until we "become more aware of how our bodies are both the metaphor and the substance of our struggle against domination" that we will be able to move towards resistance. [51] Hence the need for *education for health.*

Crawford is critical of those who unreflectively put forward the idea of education as the vehicle for the promulgation of self-care and self-responsibility for health, largely on the ground that the proponents of health education rarely address the social context in which that education should take place. [52] From this it does not follow that he is against health education. Indeed, he believes that health education programs should be encouraged. His worry is that if the content of health education is limited merely to supplying information about improving lifestyles through individual behavior modification, health education is tantamount to victim-blaming. Much of the literature on health blatantly assumes that education is a panacea for the major health problems confronting society, though little is done to exhibit clearly the manner in which education could or should actually be utilized for this purpose.

There is no doubt that health education in the limited context of teaching about health issues alone would be of little value, and we will in the next chapter see why this is so. Suffice it to say here that in the present work we distinguish between conventional health education and educating for health. We have no intention of limiting health education to conventional matters of health alone, nor do we envisage the task of health education simply as the transmission of knowledge. On the view we will propose, *education for health* is to be seen as part of a process of general awakening whereby individuals come to realize the level of their own importance in maintaining personal and community health. Through education for health as here conceived people will be made aware of the unique contribution which they as individuals can make to the health of their community, their families, and to themselves. Education for health will be directed also to political and social issues that involve people in their homes, their workplaces, and their leisure environments, as well as stressing the importance of positive health practices and the crucial link with the natural environment.

Summary

In this chapter we have seen that primary health care is emerging as the principal vehicle for the delivery of health care. Being focused in and on each local community, the services it provides depend upon its intimate and full integration with relevant contextual factors such as nutrition, sanitation, housing, peace, and work. Primary health care evolves from and reflects the economic exigencies, along with the peculiar cultural and political characteristics of the global community.

The main health problems in the community can be addressed through primary health care by the provision of promotive, preventative, curative, restorative, and supportive services according to the needs of the community or its inhabitants. Primary health care is not an isolated unit of the health care service and works through consultation with, and referral to, the central sectors of the service, to provide the most suitable care for those in the community most in need. As well as coordinating within the health sector, primary health care must connect with all related sectors that are involved in national and community development, in particular agriculture and food services, industry, education, housing, and communications.

One of the key elements of primary health care is the involvement of the community and its members in the planning, organization, and operation of the facilities required by each community to meet its needs. Primary health care makes use of local resources, including people, to the fullest extent and to this end develops through what we have called "education for health" the ability of all community members to participate.

Education is, on the view we propose, a key element in the enterprise of promoting and advancing community health. It is through participatory education that people can come to realize their ability to contribute to the development of their country and to take control of and responsibility for the health of themselves, their families and their community.

Through dialogue and discussion within the community, such education will seek to include information concerning the prevention and control of disease. The securing of safe water supplies, the monitoring of food quality and the practice of basic hygiene may also be important components in a program concerned to educate for health. Other topics such as child care, family planning, and immunization could well be included in the education syllabus. If people are to accept responsibility for their health on both a personal and a community level they will require a sound basis on which to make informed decisions about matters relating to their health. All people require education for health.

Access to health *care* is, we have suggested, a right to which all persons are entitled. It remains a reasonable observation, however, that if persons are to demand the right to health care, which includes education for health, then they do have a reciprocal responsibility to take reasonable precautions to protect and maintain their own health. The placing of responsibility on individuals should, however, not be regarded as a means of absolving other bodies, such as government or industry, from sharing the responsibility for the attainment and maintenance of health. Our intention in this regard is to help people become responsible for their health, *not* to blame them for their illness.

Health education, based on the wholistic approach, constitutes what we call "education for health" and takes into account the social, environmental, and political aspects which contribute to the health of the community. Education for health links with primary health care to allow individuals and communities to work in conjunction with health professionals to identify the environmental risks and problems associated with the health of the community. By acquiring information about such problems and the range of possible solutions, members of the community can express their informed judgement in the decision-making processes which in turn affect their physical and social environment.

Education for health rests, as does primary health care, on the premise that it is everyone's right to have a say in decisions and actions which affect them, and equally, it is thus their responsibility to exercise their rights in regard to that say. The basic commitment to the concepts of rights and responsibilities is enshrined in numerous charters and bills worldwide, and the issues which arise therein continue to be addressed by various currents of philosophical interest, because they are taken to be of fundamental importance in understanding human life. It is to this same end that the sound planning and practice of education for health is to be directed: the end, that is, of improving the quality of human life. Such planning and practice is of necessity to be established through continuing dialogue and discussion with those most affected by it, and it is part of the burden of education for health to ensure that this discussion not only takes place, but is substantively directed and well-in-formed.

CHAPTER 6

People Empowerment: Education for Health Vs Health Education

The Origins of Health Education

Formal health education began in Germany in 1792, with a course of instruction for both teachers and pupils. This course was translated into several languages, including English, and from 1798 to 1882 was a major source of health information. Throughout the nineteenth century health education in most western countries was incorporated into school programs. Dr. William Alcott wrote the first health book for children in 1829.

During the middle years of the nineteenth century, the Women's Christian Temperance Union (WCTU) had the most significant impact on health education, not only in the United States but worldwide. As James Rogers noted, "no wave of legislation having to do with school hygiene and sanitation has so swept the country as that accompanying the temperance movement." [1]

The latter years of the nineteenth century saw a dwindling in health instruction as competition increased in regard to those subjects necessary for admission to higher education at college and university level. In the U.S. it was as a result of this competition, however, that the recommendations for preparation of teachers in health instruction emerged. Edward Hartwell, in 1895, asserted:

> school hygiene as an art is concerned with the measures that science and experience have shown to be helpful and efficacious for securing the normal growth and development of pupils and the normal activity of teachers under the conditions incident to school life. . . .No mere graduate of a medical school - much less a mere normal school graduate is competent to perform the duties of a school hygienist. He should be trained in his specialty like other specialists. [2]

With the twentieth century and the emergence of *progressive* education came the increasingly popular idea that pupils are each unique individuals. The notion that education is nothing more than a social vehicle for the transmission of knowledge was called into question. Changing concepts, such as the forementioned in education, coupled with a more positive approach to hygiene in particular, led to rapid revolution in health education in most western countries. The term *health education* was proposed to replace *hygiene* in 1919 at a conference of the Child health Organization in New York. It is apparent that in the United States, at least, health education had by 1938 become an accepted, separate, and academically respected subject. However, in 1967 a study by

Mayshark concluded that the efficacy of health education programs was directly related to the individual school administrations' commitment to the idea. [3] According to this study, the quality of health education varied from school to school.

There is nothing novel in the idea that a crisis can call attention to what is lacking in a community, but it nonetheless represents a truth. The two World Wars revealed how widespread poor health was in many men conscripted into the armies of Britain and the United States. The drug crisis of the 1960s in America and later in other countries saw the introduction of drug-education classes. Acquired Immune Deficiency Syndrome in the 1980s similarly brought with it resurgence in sex and health education. Whilst in recent years the growing crisis in obesity has followed suit. It is the poor results achieved by these conventional health-education programs born out of "crisis" which demands the implementation of a new model of education for health, based not only on health issues but the relevant social, political, and environmental concerns of the global community. More than two centuries after formal health instruction began, there is still no coherent and well-articulated philosophical basis of health education. Let us see what assumptions underpin health education as we move closer to the task of articulating its philosophical foundations.

There are at least three fundamental assumptions which underline most of the contemporary programs in health education. These basic assumptions can be stated as follows: firstly, that health behaviors are mediators of health status; secondly, that health behaviors are the result of knowledge, beliefs, and attitudes; and thirdly, that specific behaviors, when changed, improve health.

These assumptions can be supported historically. For example, vaccines were tested for efficacy, and then health education programs were instituted to increase vaccination rates. Methods of preventing unwanted births were tested before the start of family-planning education. Recently, health education has turned to preventive lifestyle measures and chronic diseases. However, as Lorig and Laurin have asserted, "in these areas, based on epidemiological and other studies, changed behavior has been assumed to effect health status. However, there is little confirmation of this hypothesis from prospective experimental studies." [4] In what follows in this chapter we will consider the extent to which health education programs based on the above three assumptions and implemented in developed and developing countries have or have not been successful. Although it is to be admitted that our examination is by no means exhaustive, the studies chosen are representative of the types of health education programs in most countries in recent years. Our contention is that conventional health education, not unlike conventional medicine, has been applauded beyond its merits. Only by broadening its philosophical basis to incorporate the wholistic concept of educating for health can "health education" achieve the progress in *public* health which it seeks.

Health education and lifestyle changes

Most of the present emphasis on health education in developed countries arose out of work in the 1970s in the United States. The results of this work have been less than satisfying to health educators. Let us consider some case studies to explain why.

Possibly the largest study was the MRFIT (Multiple Risk Factor Intervention Trial), conducted in the U.S., in which twelve thousand men at risk for coronary heart disease were randomized into a "usual-care" group and a Special Intervention (SI) group receiving "stepped-care" treatment (i.e., medications of increasing strength introduced as blood pressure increased) for hypertension, counseling for smoking, and dietary advice for lowering blood cholesterol. [5] After seven years the SI group had decreased risk factors. However, no significant difference in cardiac mortality was demonstrated between the two groups.

Considerable controversy abounds concerning the reasons for these findings. What is unproblematic, however, is that, for whatever reason, the original hypothesis of the 1982 MRFIT trial that "modification of elevated serum cholesterol levels, hypertension, and cigarette smoking in persons at risk of death from heart attacks would result in reduction of coronary death rates" remained unsubstantiated. [6] Similarly, in 1977 Paffenbarger et al. [7] demonstrated an association between exercise and decreased cardiac mortality. However, in 1980 Sedgewick and his colleagues in a six-year prospective trial concluded that their results "did not support the view that classical risk factors for coronary heart disease improve with increased physical activity and fitness." [8]

In North Karelia, Finland, a ten-year community study was carried out aimed at reducing cardiac mortality by means of community-wide health education focusing largely on smoking and the intake of dietary cholesterol. In his study, the population of Kuopio, a neighboring province, was used as a control group. After five years, North Karelia had fewer smokers, and its population used less dietary cholesterol than did Kuopio. [9] Ironically, its cardiac mortality was slightly *higher* than Kuopio. After ten years, the population of North Karelia had largely maintained the changed behavior and had a 24% reduction in cardiac mortality as compared to Kuopio, which had a 21% reduction. [10] When the data were analyzed by sex, only women in North Karelia showed a significant reduction in cardiac deaths compared to the women in Kuopio, a reduction of 51% in the one case as compared with a 36% reduction in the other.

From the Karelia study therefore, it would at first blush seem reasonable to conclude that during the second five years of the study, women's changes in health behavior may have accounted for their reduction in cardiac mortality. During the same time period, however, the rate of smoking in North Karelia women actually increased by 5%. There was also a slight trend for women to use more dietary cholesterol than men. The only area where women had a more beneficial health behavior change than men was in their sugar intake. [11] Although there are many possible explanations for the seeming inconsistencies, the North Karelia project supports neither strongly nor unequivocally the argument that lifestyle changes alone are linked to changes in health status.

In a program at Brown University, Rhode Island, medical students were involved in a coronary heart disease risk-factor project. This involvement had a twofold purpose for the students. It was designed firstly to allow them to see the benefits of behavior modifications in caring for patients at risk of heart disease, and secondly to bring about lifestyle changes in the students themselves. Reporting this study in 1987, Leyden et al. concluded that although there was a reduction in the serum cholesterol level in the participating group, along with reduction in diastolic blood pressure and bodyweight, the students who chose to participate in the program were motivated by the fact that they had slightly higher levels in these variables to begin with than those students who chose not to participate in the study. [12] Among the women in the trial the repeat measurements did not differ from those who did not participate. It was suggested by the researchers that "these observations plus the fact that changes also occurred in 'non-targeted' variables imply that some of the changes may have been due to chance or to such statistical factors as regression to the mean." [13] As this project was an elective part of a required activity, and the participants were well educated and highly motivated, the modest success reported is not suggestive of good outcomes in poorly educated or less motivated people.

In 1985 Assaf et al. found in comparing three methods of teaching women how to perform breast self-examination that the use of breast models incorporated with audiovisual material and pamphlets resulted in a greater increase in knowledge and skill in examining breasts compared to methods which employed only pamphlets or audiovisual instruction. [14] The breast-model training group also reported more frequent examination of their breasts than did the other training groups. The researchers reported that the women who participated in the trials "may have been more receptive to learning breast self-examination than women in the general population" as they were drawn from a free cancer screening clinic. [15] The study only followed up the women at a short interval and so it is difficult to predict whether not only the skill of breast examination would have been retained but also the actual behavior of performing the examination on a regular basis.

In 1986 a study conducted by Flaherty et al. produced similar results in the United Kingdom when two methods of instruction for breast self-examination were compared and analyzed. [16] One group was taught the skill in a clinic situation where they were simultaneously examined by a nurse and thus reassured that they did not have any breast lumps. The other group was taught in a class setting by the same nurses who taught the clinic group. It was found that the greatest compliance with breast self-examination resulted in the group taught in the non-clinical setting, contrary to the hypothesis. The factor contributing to this variation was found to be the motivation of the non-clinic group who voluntarily came to learn about breast self-examination, rather than having it included as part of their clinic visit.

An increase in knowledge was also demonstrated following an education program regarding breast self-examination in Edinburgh. However, Roberts et al. were not able to report an increase in compliance in actually examining breasts following the program. [17] What they did find, however, was that many women do not feel particularly susceptible to breast cancer and that they were in fact more interested in material related to general health. This led Roberts and her colleagues to conclude that "promoting information about breast cancer might best be done in the context of general health." [18]

An interesting study was carried out by Gravell et al. in 1985 with an aim to examine the effect of social network communications in encouraging the discussion of breast self-examination among women. [19] The results of this study suggested that education intervention which includes explicit messages to encourage discussion with social network members is effective in increasing communication with mothers, female siblings, and friends. Furthermore, the mothers of subjects so encouraged had a higher quality of breast self-examination practice than the control group. The subjects in this trial were college students, who, like the medical students in the heart risk-factor study, come for the most part from a well-educated background; this being so, it is difficult to predict the extent to which the findings in relation to them would generalize to the overall population.

In Bangladesh, Stanton et al. found that while villagers and urban dwellers showed an increase in knowledge about sanitary measures, such as hand-washing after defecation and prior to handling food, but did not demonstrate the appropriate behaviors when observed. They concluded that, in "at least for practices related to sanitation and hygiene, the responses to questionnaires do not correlate with observed household practices." [20]

An experimental school-based health education and personal development program in the northern suburbs of Sydney reported considerable success in lifestyle changes of secondary students in respect of reduced alcohol and tobacco consumption and increased exercise. Homel et al. also reported an increase in knowledge in the secondary students, but could not substantiate this finding among the primary students in the survey. [21] Homel and his colleagues attributed much of the success of the program to the fact that "the venture was undertaken co-operatively between the Health Commission and the Education Department," thus allowing a realistic balance between health and educational expertise. [22] When studying attitudes of school children and nurses to health, Maddock et al. concluded that:

> it is apparent that "mere knowledge is not enough": that is, knowing that something is dangerous," bad for you," or more generally not conducive to well-being might not be enough to ensure appropriate behaviors (the phenomenon of the physician who smokes cigarettes is well known). [23]

Parcel and his colleagues introduced health education into preschools in a program designed to encourage healthy behaviors such as eating low-sugar snacks, brushing teeth, exercising, avoiding accidents with matches, sharp objects, or poisonous substances, and avoiding other dangerous situations. The results of this study were mixed, with the four-year-olds in the study showing improvement in safety behavior compared to the control group, though in selection of snacks they were inclined to choose those foods with a higher sugar content. The Parcel program incorporated the mothers of the children into the study as well as the children. However, they still concluded that "factors outside the school, such as home environment, and other sources of reinforcement provide role models and support of behavior which may conflict with the targeted health and safety behavior." [24] They thus recommended that school health education programs require greater parental involvement, and that consideration of other environmental aspects needs to be incorporated. The earlier study to which we referred by Homel et al. also recommended that parental involvement needed to be increased in order to encourage long-term behavior changes. [25]

According estimates, as many as 15 million Americans had participated in some kind of health education program in worksites, universities, community wellness programs, health fairs and health care organizations. [26] However, despite its persuasiveness, viewers of the literature have found little evidence for its efficacy in actually changing individual behavior. [27]

When all is said, it is clear from the foregoing studies that health education programs directed to lifestyle changes seem in most cases not to have resulted in long-term behavioral changes. In those that have had relatively long-term success, such as the North Karelia project, changes in behavior aimed at improved mortality or morbidity have been largely unsuccessful.

Health education and chronic disease

Data regarding education of patients with chronic disease has demonstrated more encouraging changes in health status alone, or in both behavior and health status. The assumption drawn from this, which forms the basis of many education programs, is that changes in behavior are associated with improved health status.

Hypertension is one of the most frequently studied areas in relation to patient education, based on the assumption that behavior change results in lowering of blood pressure. However, few studies actually present statistical evidence to support this assumption. The behavior change most commonly associated with blood-pressure control is compliance with medications.

McKenney and associates randomized fifty patients with hypertension; twenty-five received counseling from pharmacists, the remainder received the usual care. [28] A 25% increase in medication compliance was reported in the study group and the number of subjects with normal blood pressure increased by 59%. No such improvement was demonstrated in the control group.

In another study in which physicians who had been tutored to improve their effectiveness as educators were the patient instructors, medication compliance improved significantly. The number of patients with normal blood pressure was 69% as compared to 36% of patients in the study with the control physicians. [29] Nessman and colleagues also studied an intervention to increase compliance among noncompliant hypertensive patients. Patients were assigned to either a nurse-operated hypertension clinic (control) or a patient-oriented experimental group. Experimental patients had lower diastolic blood pressures and were more compliant than control patients. [30]

These three studies, while suggesting both that compliance with treatment had improved and that blood pressures were lowered, did not measure the association between behavior change and lowered blood pressure. In other words they did not comment on whether those who increased compliance were the same patients as those who lowered their blood pressures. Once again, the link between behavior change and health status has not been supported by studies undertaken to assess it.

In a study by Haynes et al. it was shown, however, that "the changes in compliance among experimental patients were paralleled by decreases in their diastolic blood pressures." [31] Although more than 50% of the control group in this study demonstrated a reduction in blood pressure, they also decreased their compliance.

In a more recent study by Morisky et. al. the use of a family health education program was implemented to support hypertensive patients. The subjects assigned to the group in which family education formed part of the management scheme showed that "improvements were evident in medication taking behavior (14%), appointment keeping behavior (80%) and weight and blood pressure control (20%)." [32] It was also reported that the long-term effects were positive in that, at two and five year follow-up, blood-pressure control, appointment keeping, and weight control were significantly improved or maintained in the family support group.

While there is no suggestion that the foregoing review of hypertension education programs is exhaustive, our survey clearly indicates that factors other than health-educational ones, both behavioral and non-behavioral, appear to influence the positive outcome for gaining control of the actual hypertension. However, as the Morisky study showed, the patient with hypertension can increase positive health behaviors when the concept of education is broadened to include family education as a component in patient education.

Studies of *diabetes* also gives several examples in which changed behaviors appear not to be associated with positive outcomes in terms of improved health status. Forty years ago in 1969 Williams concluded that "no correlation has been demonstrated between performance of the prescribed therapy and good or poor control of the disease." [33] More recently, Webb concluded similarly that "while diabetics showed significant improvements in knowledge, dietary composition and health benefits, no significant changes were observed . . . . in measures of glucose control, weight or serum cholesterol." [34]

A useful measure of the efficacy of education programs for diabetic patients is to assess the number of admissions which they require to hospital. Whitehouse et al. found that the non-attenders of an education program over a five-year period had higher rehospitalization than did the attenders. However, when hospitalizations were classified according to cause, which could be affected by education, no differences were found between the attenders and the non-attenders. Thus even though the attenders had fewer admissions to the hospital, they did not seem to be related to what was taught. These findings led the authors to state:

"Intuitively, we believe that basic diabetes education reinforced by follow up sessions does favourably influence the future of the person with diabetes, yet it is important to establish this assumption." [35]

One of the most common chronic health problems of today is *obesity*. The basis of most weight loss programs is the assumption of a correlation between reduced food intake and weight loss. Again, the associations here between changed behavior and weight loss are not always clear. In 1978 a study by Brownwell found that "correlations between total calorie scores and measures of ideal weight and weight loss were nonsignificant. Self-reported food intake did not correlate with weight loss." [36] In a study by Stalonas et al. in 1978 it was concluded that "the data indicated that our subjects engaged in the required behaviors at a reasonably high level. However, the combined influence of all behaviors accounted for a small and insignificant proportion of the weight loss variance." [37]

Whilst the most urgent challenge to nutritional health for the 21st century is addressing the epidemic of obesity, Kushner et al also found more recently that even practitioners reported little confidence in their ability to help educate their patients to change unhealthy behaviors. [38]

Arthritis is another of the most common of the chronic diseases, affecting countless millions worldwide. The relationship between health status of the persons afflicted with arthritis and behavior change is also not well-established. Liang, for instance, found no correlation between services rendered and arthritis health status in arthritis groups receiving care with and without patient advocacy services. [39] Similarly, no correlation was demonstrated between knowledge and improved family relationships in a study of support groups for arthritis sufferers, nor was there a correlation between knowledge and coping in the patients themselves. [40] Lorig and her colleagues found, in a study following an education program designed to improved self-management of pain in arthritis patients that only a weak association existed between increases in self-management behaviors, such as the practice of relaxation and exercise, and decreased pain. [41]

In 1984 Lorig and her colleagues reviewed eleven studies related to chronic disease and published in journals printed that year and found that in seven of the studies there was no association between changed health behavior and health status. In only one segment of one study was there a direct association between behavior change and health status. While admitting the limited number of studies examined, Lorig was convinced that the studies discussed were representative of health education in the field of chronic disease. [42]

Concerned to close the gap between "knowing the good" and "doing the good," [43] health educators have adapted a number of theories and models drawn from the psychology of learning on which the practice of health education has come to be based. Among those theories and models which have figured prominently in the work of health educators the following have perhaps been most influential. Expressed here in a much-truncated form they are:

1. *Social learning theory*, presented by Rotter in 1954, postulates that behaviors are a function of the expectancy of reinforcement and the value of the reinforcement. [44] Rotter's theory has been supplemented by Bandura, who

argues for the importance of antecedent social stimulus events.[45,46,47,48] More recently, Bandura has theorized that future behavior is based on one's present perception of the ability to perform the projected behavior. This latter concept is termed "self-efficacy."

2. *The Knowledge-Attitude-Practice* (KAP) model was originally designed to assist family planning programs. It hypothesizes that although increased knowledge does not in itself necessarily affect behavior, the knowledge that a person has regarding a particular health matter may serve to bring about a change in attitude which will, in turn, lead to behavior modifications related to that health matter. [49]

3. *The "health belief model"* and its many variations states that the likelihood of taking recommended preventative health action is based on:
  a. perceived susceptibility to disease,
  b. perceived threat of the disease,
  c. perceived benefits of preventive action,
  d. perceived barriers to preventive action. [50]

This model arose from an interest in trying to determine why some people use health services and other do not, and why there is a high rate of noncompliance with health and medical recommendations.

Common to all these models is the assumption that the primary goal of health education is behavior modification and that, to a greater or lesser extent, beliefs and attitudes can be shaped to mediate the desired behavioral changes. [51] Dichotomies, however, prevail in this area. Given consensus that experience is the source of learning, there remain two polarized views on the exact psychology of learning: the *stimulus-response* (SR) *associationist* and the *cognitive-field theorists.* The SR associationists believe in shaping pupil behavior by presenting sequences of stimuli and responses that lead students to the *desired* outcome. The cognitive-field theorists, on the other hand, reject the view that learning constitutes a relationship between a stimulus and a response. Instead, the cognitivists view education as involving the creative reorganization and rearrangement of previous ideas and experiences leading to new thought patterns or cognitive processes which might be called "insight."

The contemporary split is quite well elaborated in the writing of B. F. Skinner and J. Bruner. [52] Skinner advocates controlled experiences and Bruner stresses free experience. Pavlov is generally regarded as the instigator of SR associationism with his well-known experiments on dogs. He demonstrated that a physiological response would occur following an auditory stimulus suggestive of an *association* between sound and food. Following Pavlov's lead, J. B. Watson argued that psychologists should be able to rest their claims on observable behavior akin to that provided in Pavlovian experimentation, and this led to the establishment of the school now named *behaviorism.* The application of behaviorist principles to learning theory inspired the development of an early form of educational behaviorism promulgated chiefly by Thorndike. Influenced by these developments, and believing that contemporary education was inefficient, Skinner advocated programmed learning as an offshoot from the SR theory.

Cognitive-field theory developed almost simultaneously with SR theory. Although its philosophical roots extend several hundred years into the past. Comenius in the seventeenth century believed that children should learn from life, not school, or to put it differently, things at school should be learned for their value in life. Rousseau in the eighteenth century felt that education should derive from the utilization of the senses, from direct experience. He viewed individuals as "feeling hearts," not as machines to be programmed or as animals to be conditioned. Dewey's view that thinking is the essential element of education was influenced in part by Petalozzi, Froebel, and Tolstoy. Gestalt psychologists were conducting learning experiments around the same time as the SR theorists, the former equated the process of learning with the process of gaining insight. Bruner added to Dewey's "learn by doing" by advocating the "discovery approach" - arranging the learning environment to allow students to discover ideas on their own.

The SR theorists accept the basic premise that behavior results from environmental experiences and, supporting the Skinnerian view that modern education is inefficient, believe that education should decide in advance the most desirable behavior and arrange a suitable chain of experiences to produce the desired outcomes. As Skinner states: "Permissiveness is not policy; it is abandonment of policy, and its apparent advantages are illusory. To refuse to control is to leave control not to the person himself but to other parts of the social and non-social environment." [53]

Believing that controlled education encourages conformism and uniformity [54] rather than diversity, the cognitive-field theorists reject the traditional regimentation of schools. They do, however, believe that guidance is necessary to foster discovery and inquiry. It is this guidance which supplies direction to the expression of educational freedom.

Such are the very rough outlines of these two contemporary schools of thought on the psychology of education. Health educators have attempted to adapt the theory and practice of health education to one or the other as the intellectual habits of the time and place dictated. On occasion, the rational process of arbitration may also have been at work in the use made of these conflicting schools. As Dewey in 1938 reflected on the arguments of the day:

> It is the business of an intelligent theory of education to ascertain the causes for the conflicts that exist and then, instead of taking one side to the other, to indicate a plan of operations proceeding from a level deeper and more inclusive than is represented by the practices and ideals of the contending parties. [55]

More recently Hilda Taba took a similar position when she asserted:

> . . . in effect the study of psychological principles underlying curriculum and teaching is somewhat akin to an archeological expedition: one can find fossilized remains of almost any learning theory that ever existed, no matter how outdated or discredited it may be. . . . Learning is complex and there are

> many different kinds: mastering motor skills, memorizing information, learning feelings, concepts and intellectual skills, such as generalizing, scientific enquiry and problem solving. Learning theorists may be deceiving themselves by looking for common laws to explain processes which may have little in common. Such empirical laws of learning as exist are limited to the lowest levels of learning. Little as yet is known precisely about the higher levels of learning, such as thinking, attitudes and interests. [56]

Recent progressive educational theories hold that the most essential element in learning is the individual involved in that learning. This human aspect of education has been particularly strongly emphasized by some theorists. Combs, for example, succinctly expressed the commitment to humanistic education thus:

> If we want to humanize the process of learning, we must make a systematic search for things that destroy ineffective learning and remove them from the scene. If we are to humanize the process of learning we must take the student in as a partner . . . . We decide what people need to know and then we teach it to them whether they need it or not. As a result some students discover that school is a place where they study things that don't matter and drop out. [57]

Similar educational sentiments are shared by writers such as Illich, Buber, and Freire, to name only a few. On this view much of the supposed "education" that actually takes place in the name of health is irrelevant to those doing the learning, and consequently they learn poorly, as we saw in our earlier discussion of conventional health education.

It should thus be clear that health education based on education aimed at changing individual behavior will for the most part meet with only limited success.

The belief that health is a dynamic process involved in the lives of all individuals, and that all individuals are in constant interaction with their cultural and physical environment generates the need to adopt a view of health education within which the sociocultural environmental aspects of health can be considered. [58] The reconceptualization of health education, that is to say, requires an adequate contextualization of the issue of health. Any adequate model will thus encompass more than education regarding health alone and will reflect the commitment to total national development.

Frankena provides a model of education which has relevance for the implementation of a more comprehensive educational program for health. Frankena's model can be used to provide a *coherent* structuring of the issues relevant to the education debate. It will consider not only the *how* of educational practice but also the *why* and *what.* In other words it will base the praxis of education on critical reflection.

Philosophy of education for health

The Frankena model is concerned to disturb the complacency of educational practitioners who have failed to reflect on the philosophical foundations upon which they base their practice. [59]

According to Frankena, statements of basic normative belief are abstract premises which define the most general purposes of education or health education. In reference to health such statements might be that education for health *should* create a healthy global community; health is a desirable process; health is a human right; health demands human effort for its attainment and maintenance.

The second type of statements which figure in the foundational structure of education are basic factual premises, general though perhaps less abstract statements which include propositions about dispositions and the nature of personkind or knowledge or the cosmos. In relation to health such a statement might be "health is a process not a state," or "moderation in dietary intake is possible," or even "knowledge about matters of health is possible."

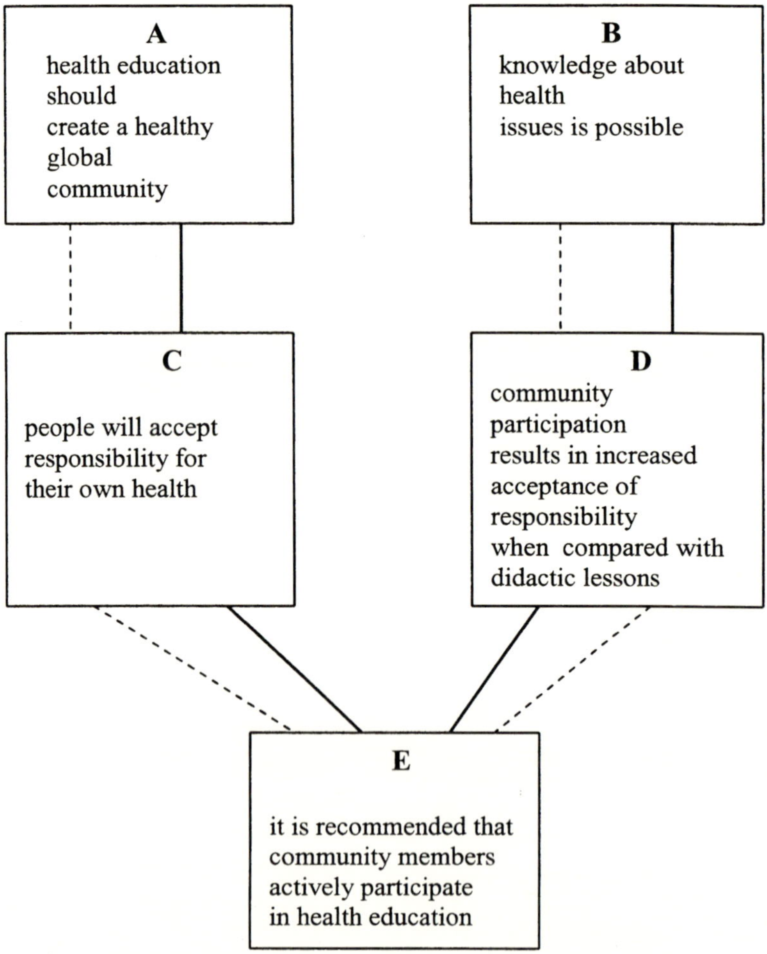

Figure 1. The Frankena Model applied to education for health.

Statements about the actual dispositions to be fostered in order that the normative premises can be realized are located in Box C of the diagrammatic model which follows in Figure 1. Box C will also include statements of aims or objectives. An example of such a statement in the context of health would be, "as a result of health education, the health status of the community will improve," or, "as a result of the anti-smoking campaign, X number of people will give up smoking," or, "as a result of the classes in preparation for parenthood, there will be a reduction in the number of child-abuse cases."

A complete theory of education, according to Frankena, will "tell us what we should do in order to acquire or foster the dispositions recommended in Box C." In other words there should be statements relating to the method and means of education, curriculum statements, administrative policy statements, and the like. Such statements will be found in Box D. These statements will be supported by factual evidence as to the worth of a particular method or approach to education, so that in the final Box E, *recommendations for practice* can be made. An example of a Box D statement in respect of health might be, "using a peer support group member as a teacher was a better method of teaching than having a doctor as the teacher." This type of statement would be expected to follow a study of an education program designed to modify the dietary habits of diabetic patients. From this the Box E statement would follow, namely, "it is recommended that peer support group members act as teachers in diabetic education programs."

In the light of this model Frankena suggests that there are three possible patterns of educational interaction. Firstly, the ABC pattern states the dispositions to be fostered and why they should be fostered (Box A), as well as the pertinent higher-order facts about personhood or knowledge (Box B), leaving the practical aspects (Box D & E) to administrators and teachers.

The second is the CDE pattern which explores *what* should be done (Box D) to foster the dispositions (Box C), giving evidence and arguments for the preference of one method over another to conclude in a particular practice directive (Box E). The third, and most significant, is of course the ABCDE pattern, which takes into account both of the other patterns and gives a comprehensive basis for the philosophy underpinning education. For this pattern to be utilized extensive cooperation and communication between the policy makers using the ABC segment of the model and the practitioners working with the CDE segment is needed. Often those doing the educating in the field lose faith in health education because of the restricted view that the CDE segment of the model gives. Without the normative and factual premises upon which to pin actual practice, the overall conception of education for health is blurred. Equally, those who work only with the ABC pattern are relatively useless to the practitioner faced by immediate and obvious health problems.

Frankena proposes a five step analysis to determine if a philosophy of education is firmly based on a complete normative philosophy, and suggests that through such analysis one can build one's own normative philosophy of education in any field.

1. One must first look to see what dispositions it says education should foster (Box C).
2. Next, one must try to determine the rationale given to show that education should foster those dispositions. To do this one must:

a. see what its basic normative premises are—its basic values, principles, or ends (Box A);

b. see what factual premises are brought in (implicitly or explicitly), empirical, theological, or philosophical (Box B);

c. see how these go together to make a line of argument of the ABC pattern to show that the dispositions listed should be cultivated.

3. Then one should look for recommendations about ways and means of teaching, administering, etc, (Box E).
4. Fourthly, one must seek to discover the rationales for these recommendations. To do this one must:

a. see what factual statements based on observation and experience are brought in - possibly borrowed from psychology, etc, (Box D).

b. see if any premises from Boxes A and B are used here.

c. see how these go together to make a line of argument (or battery of separate arguments) to show that the ways and means recommended should be used in the cultivation of dispositions listed (Pattern CDE).

5. All along, of course, one should notice any definitions or bits of analysis that occur and see how they fit into the discussion. [60]

It becomes apparent that for a sound basis to be established on which to found education for health, all five aspects (ABCDE) of the Frankena model need to be considered. Yet as was seen in the case examples given earlier in this chapter, only those aspects in boxes CDE have generally been considered. This may account for the limited success of health education programs in the past. For effective programs to be established those who determine the purposes of education for health, based ideally on the most general factual and normative premises, must also do so in conjunction with those who will, at the community level, be putting into practice the best available methods. If those who are at the interface between the community and the health services do not contribute to the formation of a model of education for health, it is unlikely that the model will be based on ways and means which are acceptable to local communities and the health workers who have the task of implementing the education programs. Consistent with the idea of individual and community involvement in primary health care is participation in the formulation of a model of education for health designed to ensure that people will gain maximum benefit from such programs.[61]

Summary

Health is a dynamic process, involving individuals not in isolation but in an interaction with other living creatures and the total environment. To focus health education on individual behavior changes is to limit the scope of education and to indulge in practices that will lead more and more to the concept of blaming the victim for his or her health deficiencies. From the studies by Gravell and Morisky which included aspects of social networking and communication, it can be seen that a broader focus of education is more likely to have positive health outcomes. By including family members in the health program, for example, individuals seem less likely to feel isolated by their disease. They also find it easier to accept that their disease, like other aspects of life, involves themselves and others in a subtle process of dynamic interaction. Similarly, the programs that encourage open discussion with other members of the social network allow health issues to be raised in the normal social environment and not cloistered away in a hospital or clinic. Health is part of everyday life; to discuss matters of health in isolation from that life is to deny the right of individuals to take responsibility for their own health. Such isolation also continues to steep not *health* but *disease* in the "mysticism of medicine." The mystification of medicine serves to foster institutional structures and behavioral patterns which make people dependent and disempowered. They are deprived of the responsibility of their own health, along with the ability to make informed choices as to which behavioral patterns are healthy and which are not.

We have seen that health education has been conducted in such a way that it attends only to conventional matters of health, leaving unattended the underlying social, political, and environmental issues which profoundly affect health.

After exploring briefly the history of health education and aspects of the debate which surrounds it, it became apparent that health education has been based on a limited model, deriving from bioreductionist medicine [62]. The debate between the stimulus-response theorists and the cognitive-field theorists, and other schools of thought, while perhaps of benefit for the practice of conventional health education, does little to establish firm ground for the development of what we called "education for health."

Past attempts at health education have been met with limited success, partly because they rely upon a model which is medically myopic and partly because the *method* of health education has itself been disruptive of autonomy [63]. The assumption has been that the educator knows best what to be taught and how best to teach it, without due consideration to the individual integrity of those being taught [64]. From this it follows that all too often the community and individuals who have been taught have had little to say about what they need to be active in the process of education itself. Once again, this practice arises from a limited view of what is involved in education for health. If the goal of health for all is to become a reality then it is necessary for a sound philosophical basis to be established on which to pin education for health. A goal on a global scale will not be realized if each separate group involved in the health care services evolves a separate and perhaps conflicting philosophy for health education.[65]

While it is of great importance that the praxis of education be developed through dialogue with each local community, or with each individual involved in education for health, it is of equal importance that the basic normative and factual premises underpinning the effort of health education be developed. Philosophers of education and health educators who have much to contribute to the A and B boxes in the Frankena model must work also in conjunction with the health workers who will be involved in the practice of health education. Between them the fuller Frankena model can be established as a functional whole, rather than as two separate decision mechanisms. This is a necessary requirement if education for health is to make an effective contribution to the goal of health for all and to assist promote "the active role of people in and with their reality." [66]

Community participation in health care and education for health provide the practical framework within which the wholistic approach to health embraced throughout this volume can be achieved. Our examination of the wholistic orientation make it clear that neither health care nor education for health is the sole prerogative of health professionals, be they traditional or so-called alternative practitioners. When all is said, it is incontestable that health care and education for health take on new and comprehensive dimensions of meaning when they are viewed within the wholistic scheme of global interconnectedness which characterizes the world in which we live. The philosophical foundations of the new global and interconnected we in which we find ourselves a part of will be elaborated on in the next chapters.

CHAPTER 7

The philosophical principles of unfolding consciousness

We begin this volume with a consideration of medicine's progressive reliance upon the reductionist tradition in science as the source of medical knowledge. As a method of medical enquiry, we saw that the reductionist disposition of science is determinately analytic: the aim is to understand the structure and function of living things by breaking them down into the fundamental parts of which they are made. Bioreductionism thus leads to the initial analysis of the human body into its anatomical, physiological, and biochemical aspects. These aspects are then subdivided into smaller and smaller subunits or processes which in turn admit of separate and more detailed analysis. The finer the detail possible, the more specialist is the discipline responsible for its description.

Preoccupied with cellular structures and physiochemical processes, the bioreductionist account of the place of the mind in the understanding of health and disease is decidedly ambiguous. Whether the mind is something separate from the body or something to be reduced to it remains unclear. What is clear on the bioreductionist model, however, is that if disease is 'real,' it is *organic*. This being so, the eradication of disease depends primarily upon organic intervention, and the locus of medical care is the individual and the physiochemical processes associated with disease. Health is seen as the absence of disease; health care equals disease care, and health education amounts to disease education. The bioreductionist model of medicine thus provides no adequate vocabulary for the phenomenon of health outside the semantics of disease.

Earlier chapters were concerned predominately to show that the crisis confronting conventional medicine results in large part from its allegiance to the reductio-mechanist tradition of science, or from what we called its foundation in "medical scientism." Although the emphasis upon the analytic approach to medical care has yielded some spectacular contributions at the level of *individual* intervention, we saw that the factors which determine the health of the *community* are not greatly affected by conventional medical intervention. We observed, for example, that in excess of 90 percent of the decline in the incidence of tuberculosis antedated the introduction in 1948 of the first effective antibiotics. The most significant factors determining health were seen to derive *not* from a knowledge of the physiochemical processes of disease but from a knowledge of the effects of the environment and lifestyle upon the human organism and other living organisms. This is in part why exponential increases in medical care expenditures have done little to advance community health. Progressively more conventional medical care – indeed even better medical care (whatever that may mean) has not produced the impressive improvements in health originally promised and expected of it. Infectious diseases, manifest in epidemic proportions during the last few centuries, have virtually disappeared, but only to be replaced by chronic and degenerative diseases such as cardiovascular disease, cancer, emphysema, chronic bronchitis, arthritis, stroke, and cirrhosis. Chronic diseases of this type are reported to account for over 80 percent of illness.

Given the emphasis of modern medicine upon the technological and specialized aspects of disease eradication, it is tempting to criticize medicine, as many of its detractors have done, for being *too scientific*. We submit that this is a temptation to be resisted. The problem is that conventional medicine is *not scientific enough*, being steeped in the bioreductionism of medical scientism. What has to be jettisoned from conventional medicine is not science but the scientism which restricts the scope of its method to narrow reductionist analysis.

In the light of the conceptual and practical difficulties surrounding the conventional medical orientation, many writers have found the transition to wholistic medicine a straightforward and easy step. This being so, the philosophical framework within which the wholistic approach offers a viable alternative to conventional medicine has been neglected and remains unarticulated. Much of the emerging vocabulary of the wholistic medical model has thus been relegated to the domain of rhetoric and hortatory generalization. Commenting on wholistic medicine, Glymour and Stalker write:

> "Having no tenable thesis of any interest, the wholistic advocate states a claim that is perfect banality and hopes the reader will draw a sweeping conclusion that is completely unwarranted. It is a tactic used throughout the literature on wholistic medicine" [1]

And they add:

> "However, wholistic medicine is not a scientific tradition. It has no paradigmatic work, no recognized set of problems, and no shared standards for what constitutes a solution to those problems; it also lacks the critical exchange among its practitioners that is characteristic of the sciences. Cranks have been common throughout the history of science, as Kuhn, a distinguished historian of science, knew well. The work of cranks does not constitute a scientific revolution, and no cranks appear among Kuhn's many examples" [2]

Although the objections raised by Glymour and Stalker betray the very philosophical myopia and dependence upon the medical scientism against which we have here been inveighing, certain of their misapprehensions about wholistic medicine arise from the fact that the philosophical foundations upon which it rests have not been satisfactorily enunciated. Nor can the wholistic approach to health education be fully appreciated until these foundations are laid. We accept that this is a deficiency in the wholistic approach to health, and we will in the present chapter endeavor to remedy it.

Commenting on what they regard as the obscure connection between the philosophy of modern physics and medical wholism, Stalker and Glymour cite Fritzof Capra as the *doyen* or quantum holists. Capra is quoted as saying:

> ....while biomedical scientists elaborated mechanistic models of health and illness, the conceptual basis of their science was shattered by dramatic developments in atomic and subatomic physics, which clearly revealed the limitations of the mechanistic world view and led to an organic and ecological conception of reality....
>
> The conceptual revolution in modern physics foreshadows an imminent revolution in all the sciences and a profound transformation of our world view and value.
>
> Quantum theory thus reveals a basic oneness of the universe. It shows that we cannot decompose the world into independently existing smaller units. [3]

Citing another example of what they condemn as wholistic rhetoric, they refer to Larry Dossey, who writes:

> ...human consciousness and the physical world cannot be regarded as distinct, separate entities. What we call physical reality, the external world, is shaped – to some extent – by human thought. [4]

And in another quoted passage:

> Molecular theories of disease causation are now seen in a different way that in the traditional biomedical model. For we recognize in the new view that isolated derangements at the level of the atoms simply do not occur. The modern rule is that all information is everywhere transmitted. Crisp causal events that were once thought to characterize each and every human disease fade into endless reverberated chains of happenings. In the new view we see the molecular theory of disease causation as an outmoded, picturesque description. Discrete causes never occur in individual bodies because of the simple reason that discrete individual bodies do not themselves exist. [5]

Stalker and Glymour regard these passages as a sampler of three themes intertwined repeatedly in wholistic writings: one about reductionism, onc about consciousness, and one about causality. Commenting on these themes they write:

> (1) The holists have no understanding of the scientific process; their claims about the structure of contemporary and recent physical science, and the conclusions that can reasonably be drawn from that science are false and absurd. (2) There is no alternative wholistic paradigm for scientific medicine. There is only an insistence on abandoning every feature of scientific medicine, including experimental controls and experimental design generally, careful statistical analysis, use of the best relevant conclusions drawn from other sciences, and the practice of rational criticism and response to arguments. [6]

Stalker and Glymour complain that the misuse of quantum physics is not really regarded as a problem by the holists, for their ulterior motive is simply "to establish their credentials on the cheap." [7] According to Stalker and Glymour, the holists' association with quantum mechanics is not genuinely philosophical at all. Holists are interested merely in substituting conjecture and rhetoric about frontier sciences as a way of legitimating their own enterprise without satisfying the canons of rationality which define legitimate science.

Because detractors of wholistic medicine such as Stalker and Glymour define rationality by reference to the scientism which we in this book are concerned to repudiate, it is difficult to see how anything that could be said in defence of wholism (which is not itself analytic) is anything which they would find convincing. Conventional medicine is not, on the view we hold, more rational than wholistic medicine; it is merely more analytical. Moreover, if the canons of rationality involving evidence and testing which they insist on applying to wholistic medicine were applied systematically to conventional medicine, the latter enterprise would have to be deemed as irrational and unfounded as the former. Since the objections to wholistic medicine on the ground that it does not admit of the objective assessments of evidence and reason appropriate to science are not uncommon, it may be apposite to dispel the confusions which persist in this regard.

Scientism in medicine: On challenging the bioreductionist model

The relationship between medicine and religion, between health and virtue has – as we saw earlier – vacillated throughout history. In defecting from religion to science, medicine has had opportunity to advertise its apostasy as a form of enlightenment, and we have observed that Stalker and Glymour are staunch advocates of this tradition. Notwithstanding their attack on wholism, the temptation has been to think that medical science has legitimized medicine, transforming its practitioners into technological giants, the high priests of the modern church of medicine. That medicine has defected from religion to science may well have served to liberate medicine from inappropriate religious dogmas, but we have seen that the extent of its dependence upon the bioreductionist science of liberation has proved to be an allegiance to *scientism* which is itself dogmatic and blinding. The achievements of medical technology are impressive, but the technological giants of medicine are in an important sense blinded giants. Let us see why.

It is not a theory within conventional medicine that specific diseases have specific causes; this basic proposition is a fundamental tenet of reductionist medicine. The theory and practice of medicine thus rests upon certain assumptions, purportedly scientific assumptions about the organization and proper investigation of the world. In this sense, the scope and limits of medicine are to some extent circumscribed by the philosophy of reductionist science. Although reductionist science reflects the dominant image of science, the dogmatic catechism it propagates is more a matter of *scientism* than of the open enquiry of science. Scientism in medicine trades on a distinction between science and non-science by way of which medicine becomes respectable by being respectably scientific. By making the objectivity of science the prerogative of medicine, the objectivity of medicine becomes a monopoly of science.

By the turn of the twentieth century the natural sciences had become so firmly established that the inclination to generalize and to extend the reductionist approach into an all-embracing worldview could no longer be resisted. The predilection for observation and experiment was exalted and the dominant image of science as the sole arbiter of truth was crystallized. That the character of science was observational exploited the commonsense belief that *seeing is believing* and secured the view that an isomorphic relation between the hypotheses of science and the facts they depicted could be realized. For natural science to be possible – it was supposed – the world must have a certain character. Natural science is possible because it is actual; therefore the world can be ascribed the logical character which natural science presupposes as the condition of its possibility. [8] Reductionist epistemology is thus affirmed as the epistemology of science.

But what sort of character would constitute nature as a possible object of natural science? One of the most influential answers was contained in the reductionist philosophy of Ludwig Wittgenstein's *Tractatus Logico-Philosophicus*, and it was the Logical Positivists who found it there. The world, Wittgenstein said, was the totality of facts. A simple suggestion, one might think, but its simplicity was supplemented by a sophisticated logical apparatus by reference to which it was elaborated and amplified. The result was a highly complicated account of language and the world which presumed a strict isomorphism between specific linguistic items and the atomic objects to which they corresponded. A philosophical thesis thus provided the formalization of a metaphysical presumption about the possibility of science. If one grants that the world is constituted of facts, somehow 'out there' awaiting discovery and collection by any normally sighted observer with an impartial mind, science can be regarded as a neutral mechanism for cataloguing facts. Knowledge derives from experience, and it is the task of science to systematize the observational procedures which do no more than record the undiluted observational or sensory data which serve to identify the facts. Science comes to be regarded as the edifice of knowledge built upon an experiential foundation whose elements are the facts of the world.

It is to be admitted, however, that science must be something more than a systematized observational technique for fact-monitoring. For there is still the logical hiatus between this observational procedure and the experimental framework that underpinned its invention. To bring this out let us examine the role allegedly played by experimentation in the dominant image of science. Experimentation refers to the mechanisms in virtue of which we test our observations to ascertain the appropriate correspondence between the language in which they are recorded and the facts they purport to record.

One important philosophical impetus for the formalization of the experimental component derived from the correspondence theory of truth unpacked in "truth-conditional terms." The position can be set out roughly as follows: a sentence is true if whatever it asserts to be the case is the case; moreover, we determine both *what* it asserts and *whether* what it asserts is the case by determining the conditions under which it would be true. On the truth-conditional account, the instantiation of a relevant condition necessitates the exclusion of a correlative possibility. So the conditions under which it would be true to assert "the cat is on the mat" are precisely the conditions whose exclusion would render it false. Every assertion is tantamount to a denial. The possibilities it shuts out are defined by the possibilities it shuts in, and these in turn mark the conditions under which it would be true. The absence of the truth-conditions necessary for the sentence's affirmation serve as a sufficient condition for its denial. This being so, the general predilection for experimentation can be viewed as the general predilection for truth. Experiment shows the degree to which a given hypothesis or theory agrees with the undiluted observational data, and the experimental procedure becomes a verificatory procedure.

We are now in a position to delineate the components which feature in the dominant image of science and the reductionist epistemology deriving from it. There is, first, the notion that the world is constituted of facts, our sensory faculties simply monitoring the basic observational data which the world provides. There is, secondly, the notion that from the generalization of particular facts emerge general theories of laws in virtue of which prediction and explanation derive. The truth of specific explanation and predictions depends not only upon the undiluted observational data from which they derive, but also upon the verificatory procedures in terms of which they are substantiated. This is of course an epistemic, not an ontic judgment. It is not as much that verification or the failure of falsification makes a hypothesis true, as that if a hypothesis is true, it must admit either verification or failure of falsification. Although the actual mechanisms of confirmation procedure are considerably more complex than this caricature of them, the caricature preserves what is basic to the more sophisticated framework of complication. It is the verificatory procedures of science and the observational foundation which has guided their construction that conjointly serve to establish science in its dominant position of epistemic priority. The traditional view is that the judgments of science are reliable because they have been tested. That scientific claims have been corroborated guarantees, so the story goes, the supremacy of science over its unscientific competitors. By adopting the epistemology of science, medicine becomes a branch of science presumed – like the reductionism on which it is modeled – to have a monopoly on truth.

Theory-ladenness and testability

The time has now come to assess the philosophical warrant for the reductionist epistemology against which Stalker and Glymour would have us measure the rational strength of wholism. Let us first consider what many would still regard as the uncontroversial conception of "fact." If it were not for those who proceed as if *there are*, one would have supposed that sufficient work has already been done in a number of disciplines to show that *there are not* such things as *bare facts*. It is not our intention to spend much time rehearsing what are by now familiar points, but as our argument is a cumulative one, it is necessary to remind the reader of what may already be a familiar point. Any attempt to characterize reality, to specify the "facts," requires a language or symbolic system whose unit of significance is the "concept." Concepts, however, are not dictated unequivocally by the reality which stimulates and shapes them. Reality's contribution to our interpretation of it is flexible; the world does not present itself as a datum of apprehension fixed once and for all. This is why recalcitrant items of translation between language schemes reflect the extent to which different natural languages are really different ways of conceptualizing the world. This means that there are limits, logical limits to what can be said in a particular language, so that the range of possible concepts conditions and delimits the range of possible facts. A scientific theory is thus not given to us ready-made by the data of observation. What we regard as a fact is itself determined by the language in which it is expressed as a fact. There is no undiluted observation independent of the language; there are only observations reported in observation languages. The very language in which our observations are reported is in turn conditioned by prior theories. In this respect there are no raw or uninterpreted data. Even mensurability and the numerical values it licenses depend upon theoretical assumptions more comprehensive than the procedures of measurement incorporated in them. That mass is an intrinsic and invariable property of a body is a "factual assumption" borne out by Newtonian mechanics. Within the universe of relativity theory the ascription of properties to a mass is relativized in such a way that the whole notion of property invariance remains empirically unattached. The point is that what we count as a fact will depend upon the universe of discourse in which the enumeration of fact obtains. [9] It is not as if a neutral observation language is available to us which transcends the theoretical framework within which a particular observation or set of observations admits of definition.

There is an informal counterpart to the formality of the theory-ladenness thesis and its treatment will be apposite here. The idea that the world is the totality of facts gives rise to the commonplace view that "seeing is believing." A more cautious statement of the position is that we should believe nothing of what we hear and only half of what we see. What we are not told, however, is how we know which half to believe. The difficulty is that the history of science is rife with examples which show that seeing is as much a matter of believing as believing is a matter of seeing. Consider, for instance, the difficulties surrounding the confirmation of the existence of the planet Neptune. In the early nineteenth century astronomers were worried by the anomalous orbit of the planet Uranus, whose orbital coordinates were clearly inconsistent with those predictions sustained by the mathematics of Newtonian gravitation. In the face of conflicting evidence, the astronomers Leverier and Adams postulated the existence of the then unknown and *unseen* planet Neptune, as a way of accommodating the discrepant data. Before the planet was actually first sighted by Galle, a number of astronomers reported having seen the planet, though their descriptions make plain that it could not have been Neptune or for that matter any other planet that they saw. In 1846 James Challis set himself the task of confirming the Neptune-hypothesis, though he did not consider it true. Believing the hypothesis false, it was only after considerable effort and numerous attempts that Challis later admitted to having unwittingly sighted the planet, having dismissed what he first saw as something other than what he knew he would have to see were the hypothesis true. The example is perhaps better assimilated to the "not-believing is not seeing" category, but this only strengthens rather than weakens the case against undiluted observation and bare fact.

It is clear that there is more to seeing than meets the eyeball; to see is to interpret. Seeing is not passive reception; it is an active exercise in problem-solving. What we regard as "the facts" depends upon the way in which our language, belief-commitments, expectations, and sensory apparatus contribute to our conceptual patterns of organization. The virginity of the eye is not something we have lost over the years; there has just never been such a thing. No eye is conceptually innocent.

We are now in a position to assess the second component in the chain of reasoning traditionally used to affirm reductionist epistemology as the preferred methodology. Science has proven itself, so the claim runs; its procedure of testability ensures the reliability of its hypotheses that survive the test. That a hypothesis has withstood our attempts to falsify it seems a strong ground for preferring it to a hypothesis which has not been tested or to one which has, but has proven unsuccessful. There is an initial plausibility in all this; indeed, it would seem counterintuitive to deny it. But there are truths which are counterintuitive, and in their light the initial plausibility of the testability inference vanishes upon inspection.

It is clear that while we rely upon the testability criterion as a guide to credibility, no acceptable statement of the criterion has ever been articulated. If one opts for a verifiability criterion, the conditions of testability would disallow universal generalizations of exhaustive scope such as scientific laws and certain hypotheses. As the quantifier ranges over an infinite domain, no finite regimentation will suffice. That all observed swans are white does not, philosophers are now painfully aware, preclude the possibility that the swan to be observed next will be not-white.

Against this it might be objected that this difficulty can easily be overcome by adopting a falsifiability criterion. It is evident, for example, that universal generalizations are susceptible of falsification. While we will later show that this judgment is not as evident as one might think, the standard reply is that the falsifiability criterion is no logical panacea. The difficulty is that while falsifiability may serve to test universal generalizations, it disallows all existential statements. The falsity of "There exists at least one unicorn" cannot be derived from any finite class of observation statements. Our failure thus far to discover any unicorns does not entail that there are none to be found, nor indeed, that we will not find one. Popperians have argued that the exclusion is innocuous, for the only statements science needs to preserve is the class of scientific laws and hypotheses which feature as the basis of explanation and prediction. Although we find it hard to fathom how science could do without testing its purely existential statements, it would be extraneous to our present consideration to contest this point here.

Notwithstanding this concession, however, the falsifiability criterion is self-stultifying. The conditions of its consistent application undermine the conditions of its reliability. Falsifiability, in any case, flouts what might be called the logical principle of propositional or truth-value symmetry. The point is simple enough, though it has been either neglected or missed by most of those who have defended falsifiability. The difficulty is that falsification of a universal generalization entails its denial, but the denial of a universal generalization is logically equivalent to asserting a purely existential statement. We could thus falsify the negative universal "Nothing has the property of being a unicorn," though the falsity of its denial, "There exists as least one unicorn," would not follow from any finite class of observation statements. We thus have a failure of parity of truth-value, as the falsifiability criterion licenses asymmetrical distributions of truth-value to statements which are logically equivalent. We can hold onto falsifiability but only at the cost of violating a fundamental law of logic: namely, if a proposition P is true, then not-P is false, and if P is false, than not-P is true.

But let us suppose that by some feat of conceptual prestidigitation we could dispel our qualms about the exact formulation of a criterion of testability. The problem is that the relation between experience and the hypothesis to be tested will itself be problematic. For it would be a mistake to think that discordant data will serve, or indeed should unqualifiedly serve always to falsify a hypothesis. One reason for this peculiar resistance to falsification involves the way in which hypothesis intermesh in complicated truth-value patterns providing the measure of the theory they constitute. As Quine has taught us, a theory might most profitably be represented as a web of beliefs, a collocation of hypotheses which correspond to reality not as individual isomorphs, but as a collective relation.[10] The total web of belief or theory is thus underdetermined by the tribunal of experience, since the collective nature of the system of belief affords a variety of internal revisions in the face of discordant data. There is considerable latitude regarding the way in which the discrepant experience distributes over the entire network of hypotheses, and the strain of discordant data is borne by readjusting the truth-value considerations which influence the equilibrium of the total belief system. On this view virtually any hypothesis can be held true, even in the face of conflicting evidence, if sufficiently radical adjustments are made elsewhere in the system.

The consequence of all this is that the falsity of a particular hypothesis is not guaranteed by observational data which conflict with the expectations characteristic of the hypothesis. An interesting example of the character of hypothesis-intermeshing is provided by K. Klein in his book *Positivism and Christianity*.[11] Klein points out that our general belief in the continued existence of the stars that form the constellation Orion is not falsified simply because of the disappearance of that constellation from the skies of the far-northern hemisphere during the summer months. The conflicting evidence is explicated by appeal to a separate hypothesis, the earth's axial tilt, which in turn supplies the prediction that that constellation will appear during the summer months in the skies of the southern hemisphere. Oddly enough, however, the hypothesis of the earth's axial tilt needs to be supplemented by yet another hypothesis, the heliocentric hypothesis, which in its turn serves to yield this last prediction.

What we see here is something of the complex manner in which a conjunction of hypotheses is amalgamated and consolidated into a theory. Recalcitrant observational data may rationally oblige internal adjustments, but such adjustments are essentially rational measures for avoiding falsification. Discrepant experimental data may reflect a failure of truth in one of the conjunction of hypotheses constituting the theory, but as the boundary conditions of a theory are not unequivocally determined by experience, one cannot always deduce from the data alone which of the constituent hypotheses is false. There is thus a process of relatively continual re-evaluation of the logical connections between the constituent hypotheses, but the process of adjustment should not be assimilated to a falsification rubric. It is not as if particular hypotheses can be lined up with particular experiences in virtue of which they are determined to be truth-carrying. The unit of cognitive significance has shifted from the hypothesis to the theory. This being so, the role which falsification actually plays in science must be far less than is claimed for it.

Again, the history of science abounds with examples that demonstrate that resistance to falsification is part and parcel of the scientific methodology. The scientist, like nearly everyone else, assumes a principle of tenacity which dictates a certain level of conceptual resilience in the face of conflicting evidence. If the scientist consistently relinquished a hypothesis whenever it conflicted with experimental observations, it would be virtually impossible to formulate constructive theories of even the simplest kind. A classic instance of the importance of the principle of tenacity emerged in the context of quantum investigations concerning beta-decay of the nucleus. The main problem was that experimental data relating to beta-decay ran contrary to the expectations logically associated with the law of conservation of energy. The experimental results were consistent, but rather than relinquish the law of conservation of energy, an auxiliary hypothesis was introduced to accommodate the discrepancy. The auxiliary hypothesis in this case marked the postulation of the neutrino, though at the time there was no independent evidence for its existence.

Contrary to much of the conventional wisdom about science, testability is not a concept sufficiently delineated to distinguish science from non-science, or the objective from the subjective. Indeed, the two seem more closely connected than many philosophers of science have traditionally supposed. Feyerabend is one philosopher who has challenged the assumption that the results of science have been achieved with incorporating what would be regarded as nonscientific elements. Without making use of the unscientific reasonings of Philolaus concerning the character of circular motion, Copernicus, for example, could not have advanced modern astronomy in the way in which he did. Feyerabend points out while astronomy reaped significant benefits from Pythagoreanism, medicine clearly profited from herbalism, wandering druggists, witches, and wise man. [12] By reverting to ideas which at the time were viewed as primitive, Paracelsus was able to make significant contributions to medicine.

Enough has now been said to suggest that the reductionist foundations of medical science are not nearly as firm as Stalker and Glymour would have us believe. We have seen that the concept of "fact" as a reductionist construct is as problematic as is the assumption that testability procedures are in themselves sufficient to ensure that science fares better than all its competitors. This assumption is part of the myth of science, and its rendering in reductionist terms is part of the dogma of scientism.

What we have seen is that science is not metaphysically neutral and that reductionist science has no monopoly on the objective investigation of disease. Indeed, the very concept of objectivity and the criteria for its ascription rest upon foundational factors which defy description in purely reductionist terms. We have observed that conventional medicine proceeds on the assumption that every disease has a cause; it is characteristic of the enterprise of pathology, for example, that pathologists trace the causes of particular diseases to the microorganisms which give rise to them. The causal principle itself, however, is not a proposition which the pathologist is concerned to establish by appeal to evidence and test. The medical researcher does not test the causal proposition in evidential terms, that is to say, for it is the concept of causality which constitutes the rationale for medical testing. If some particular disease, say cancer, does not admit of a cure, the pathologist does not conclude that the implicit belief in causal connections between diseases and their genesis is mistaken. The pathologist could relinquish many beliefs and still be properly said to be doing pathology, but the causal presupposition is not one of them. In this case, giving up one's belief in causal connections would amount to giving up one's belief in conventional pathology. This is the sense in which one might speak of "causality" as a constitutive concept, and it explains why medical reductionism is more *scientistic* than *scientific*.

Epistemic primitives and the paradox of rationality

Despite persistent protestations to the contrary, the foundations of science are not built on the virtues of "evidence" and "test" so fervently espoused by Stalker and Glymour. The foundations of science *rest upon faith*; upon beliefs which defy the evidential assessments appropriate to the beliefs which derive from them and in respect of which there is evidence. While knowledge claims are justified, certain of our beliefs are not. For there comes a point in our reasoning at which one finds propositions for which no further grounds can be supplied beyond the actual occurrence of the data which they are supposed to monitor. In putting the matter in this way it might appear as if there are no grounds which could be provided for the beliefs in this very special class. Such a judgment would be clearly mistaken. It is not so much that there can be no grounds for any of this special class of beliefs, but rather that the grounds which could be adduced in support of any of these beliefs would not be more certain than the belief itself. Recognition of this point makes it easier to appreciate that there need not be anything rationally suspect in the fact that scientists are not prepared to relinquish these beliefs in the face of specific evidence to the contrary. As Wittgenstein is reported to have said:

> I might refuse to regard anything as *evidence* that there isn't a tree. If I were to walk over to it and to feel nothing at all, I might say that I was *then* deluded, not that I was previously mistaken in thinking it a tree. If I say that I would not *call* anything "evidence" against that's being a tree, then I am not making a psychological prediction – but a *logical* statement.[13]

While the belief that there is a tree under which I am now shading myself from the sun is not arrived at by any form of inference, and though I should not regard any evidence as a disconfirmation of it, my belief need not be unreasonable. On the contrary, it could well be that to question it would be unreasonable. At the basis of well-founded belief is belief that is not founded. It is not epistemologically possible to doubt everything at once. Even doubt must rest on belief.[14]

Coming to see this is partly a matter of being re-educated to see what we have always seen, but in a different way. In learning about science we have swallowed along with what we have learned the assumptions which make science possible and intelligible. We have learned, for example, that under certain conditions we will observe that water will boil at 100ºC. What assumptions have we swallowed in learning this? Clearly, we assume that reliability of our senses; we assume that our senses are not deceiving us. This reliance upon our senses is of fundamental importance to every observational judgment made within science, but how could we establish scientifically that our senses are not deceiving us? Whatever experiment we could perform would rely upon our senses for its performance or interpretation. We cannot establish evidentially that our senses are not deceiving us, since our reliance upon our senses is itself a *condition of evidence*. The concept of evidence within science presupposes the reliability of our sensory faculties; a belief in the reliability of our senses is primitive in respect of a belief in the reliability of evidence, the latter belief being parasitic upon the former. The reason for this is logical, not psychological. It is a conceptual requirement governing the intelligent employment of the terms "evidence" and "proof." Not even science can prove something to someone who will accept nothing as proved. "Proof" presupposes that there are certain beliefs which are not themselves part of what is provable, but which give the concept of provability its sense. The foundations of science rest not upon such things as evidence and proof, but upon the constellation of beliefs, themselves neither evidence nor proven, in terms of which evidence and proof get their point within science. The same is true of knowledge.

Imagine that some putative proposition is advanced as a claim to knowledge. How would we establish that it is known? What method, that is to say, is there within science for establishing an entitlement to knowledge? The scientific method is the method of exhibiting appropriate evidential connections between the candidate knowledge-claim and the proposition(s) brought forward in evidence of it. Suppose then that some evidential proposition *e* is adduced in favor of the claim to knowledge *k*. The supporting proposition *e*, however, must itself be supported if it is to stand in an evidential relation to *k*. Once this is granted, we have the same problem securing the validity of *e* by ascertaining the requisite evidential relations which permit its acceptability, and so the study of evidential relations would seem to proceed *ad infinitum* or *ad nauseam*, depending upon one's stomach for such matters. If the epistemology of science were structured in foundational terms such as these, however, it is difficult to see how anything other than scepticism would follow. Nothing could be known if no evidential connection could be ultimately evidenced.

Rather than pursue the difficulties of the "evidential account" of the foundations of science, we urge that science has rational but not evidential foundations. Let us revert to our earlier discussion concerning the concept of proof, namely, that one cannot prove anything to someone who will accept nothing as proved. In the context of the skepticism under consideration, the extension of this view is that one can doubt everything, but not everything at once. Rational doubt presupposes that some beliefs are exempt from doubt. It would make no sense, for example, if one were to doubt that the words used to formulate the expression of doubt could be meant in the way in which they would have to be meant. Similarly, the evidential chain of reasoning *cannot* go on *ad infinitum*, otherwise the very concept of evidence would lose its point. In any chain of evidential reasoning, be it science or medicine, there comes a point at which the evidence adduced either for or against a belief will be less firmly entrenched within the entire framework of belief than the belief in question. Beliefs of this logical kind are elsewhere called "epistemic primitives." Thus, no proposition which could be alleged as an evidential support for an epistemic primitive will figure as securely in epistemic terms as does the primitive itself.

The reason for the position of epistemic priority enjoyed by primitives is that they are foundational *not* in the sense that they are the ultimate pillars of evidence, but rather in the sense that it is they which determine *what we count as evidence*. Epistemic primitives form part of the framework within which the concept of evidence gets its point, determining the hierarchy of logical relations that characterize the nature of a test. Imagine, for instance, that upon waking, one looked into the mirror and saw two bodies not one. What would one *doubt* – the veracity of one's sight or the belief that one has only one body? What serves as evidence for what? [15]

It is clear that our reliance upon sight in this case would be to rely upon that faculty of cognitive judgment associated with having one body only, and that is precisely what the judgment of sight would oblige us to concede. The conditions under which the judgment of sight could be true would in this sense undermine the conditions of its reliability. It is one's belief in bodily unity that determines the way in which contrary judgments of sight will function evidentially. One is not more certain after than before one looked that one has one body only. The belief in bodily unity is epistemically primitive in respect of the evidence adduced for or against it. We cannot – in the required sense – subject an epistemic primitive to the test, for it is itself a *condition of testability*. It is what must be accepted to test in the way in which we do, for whenever we carry out a test, we do so on the basis of certain beliefs which we exempt from test, precisely because their acceptance makes concept of a test intelligible.

This is why epistemic primitives also function as "constitutive concepts." The foundational role they play within the belief system determines the nature of the enterprise in which one is engaged. The unevidenced primitives of science have been used within scientism to determine a reductionist hierarchy, admitting of causal connections, either isomorphically or probabilistically referenced, solely in empirical terms. Epistemic primitives are constitutive, then, in the sense of featuring as organizing principles of a metaphysical kind. They provide the link between our language and our world by determining the construction we place upon the conceptual system in terms of which the world is mediated for us via our language. Our apprehension of that world is not something independent of our conceptualization of it, and inasmuch as that world does not dictate unequivocally the conceptual patterns we impose upon it, our epistemic primitives reflect on the one hand the physics of knowledge and on the other, the metaphysics of knowledge.

Medical scientism as a social phenomenon

In the light of the foregoing epistemological analysis, it should be clear that the supremacy of scientism in contemporary society and its dominance within conventional medicine is not a result of its having a monopoly on medical enlightenment and the nature of disease. The dominance of reductionist science and the attitudes it has engendered within medicine have, on the contrary, become self-serving expressions of scientism. The rejection of non-scientific (i.e., nonreductionistic) or alternate forms of medicine on the ground that they are not analytic amounts to little more than dogmatic asseverations of a self-fulfilling prophecy. In the midst of scientific enlightenment, the reductionist vision of the process of health and healing has become myopic. Reductionist science has been crystallized into metaphysics of empiricist medicine.

The pervasiveness of the scientific idiom within medicine and the sphere of its influence in health education are undeniable. We strive to make medical research scientific because we believe that its being so makes it more reliable and important than if it were not. "Science" has become a banner word, an accolade ascribed to allegedly successful aspirants for knowledge. Within our universities the Faculty of Science is no longer just one faculty among many; in this era of the self-avowed scientist, the rationality of science has become the measure of all faculties that are deemed to be worth having, including the Faculty of Medicine. To be engaged in scientific enquiry oneself, or to be associated closely with those who are, has become a status symbol. In a milieu of convoluted scientific imperialism it is no surprise that science has partisans everywhere. One need only canvass the names of various university departments to discern the extent to which the cultural domination of science has shaped our perception of ourselves and of what makes our research academically acceptable. The aegis of the natural or physical sciences has been palpably extended to include engineering science, computer science, and animal science. The proliferation of partisan terminology is further exemplified by discipline designations ranging from political and behavioral science to the social and medical sciences.

The impetus to scientific conformity within medicine has not been without its benefits, but our acquaintance with these is not in question; indeed, it is a feature of the cultural dominance of science that this should be so. Admittedly, we have in recent years become aware of some of the more undesirable side-effects of bioreductionist technology, as we have been forced to grapple with the reality of a rapidly declining environment or the medical side-effects of technological therapies and drugs. But the exercise has in an important sense been self-limiting. For it has really been the reductionist who has identified the problems of medicine, and where this has not been so, it has almost always been the scientist who has pronounced upon their resolution. That this problem solving orientation is seen by some as unexceptionable is itself a measure of the philosophical problems we are here exploring. Scientism has become self-perpetuating, furthering its dominance by capitalizing on the very objections that might otherwise have served to call it in question. As we indicated earlier, the "technological fallacy" is underpinned by the notion that improved technology will make everything better, including the things which improved technology is by its very nature bound to make worse. The standard treatment is irrelevant, treating only symptoms and leaving the deeper etiology of this conceptual disease unattended. As long as medical amelioration is defined in scientific terms which are reductionistic, conventional medicine will remain an incomplete approach to health care.

Medical scientism and dogmatism

These deliberations clearly have serious ramifications for any system of health education which pretends to do more than guarantee that society is able to perpetuate its vested institutional interests in the name of health. By assimilating reductionist science as an all-embracing worldview, the current educational approach has for the most part reflected partisan interests. Health education, not unlike general education itself, has become "intellectually sectarian." Let us now endeavor to explain this.

Because we have earlier intimated the possibility of a role within health education for spiritual or humanistic concerns of a wholistic kind, it is tempting to think that we see a place in medicine for dogmatic religion. On the contrary, our objection to dogmatic science or scientism is an objection equally to dogmatic religion. Neither has the power to emancipate the intellect from the conceptual structures which each requires for the generation of open-minded enquiry. Both dogmatic science and dogmatic religion constrict rather than enlarge the domain of intellectual freedom. Dogmas set authoritarian limits, *not logical limits*, to what it is permissible to think. To this extent dogmatic science and dogmatic religion close minds, and a closed mind represents a paralysis of imagination and the demise of education.

Most of us find it easy to conceive of dogmatic religion, but what, one might ask, is dogmatic science? Is not science by its very nature liberating? The answer to this is not easy, for there is a radical ambiguity in the use which the term "science" has. It is true that science has played an important historical role in breaking the comprehensive hold which religion once had over the mind. It has accomplished this admirable task by affording the opportunity of thinking about the world in ways other than those which had become ideologically entrenched in the institutional church. This entrenchment meant that the received wisdom was institutionalized as a vested interest of those in power. One's identity was itself tied to the institutional form in which it was made manifest. To challenge an accepted belief was therefore to challenge the institution and, by implication, those who had vested interests in its perpetuation. The reification of religion was thus expressed as a bureaucratic or institutional representation of truth. Any challenge to the institution, or to the bureaucracy that ensured its function, was registered as an objection to truth, and the objectors were maligned as heretics. The science of the time obliged a questioning of inherited beliefs and undermined the authoritarianism of the monolithic conceptual structure that had been built in the name of God. One can thus appreciate how the terms "science" and "enlightenment" came to be used coextensively. Science began as a heresy, but the reflective mode it stimulated was heresy of enlightenment.

It is crucial to recognize, however, that the equivalence between science and enlightenment is an equivalence of process, not an equivalence of content. What was enlightening about science, we suggest, was not so much the specific content of its doctrines, as that its doctrines forced reflection upon the corpus of inherited beliefs. That this is so is borne out by our earlier remarks on testability. Despite protestations to the contrary, the methodology of reductionist science is not guaranteed by its reductionist methods of knowledge acquisition. A hypothesis which has thus far survived all our tests may be rejected in the light of future experience, and similarly, a hypothesis which is degenerate and failed our tests may tomorrow be reinstated. Epistemologically speaking, the content of reductionist science is no more secure than the content of dogmatic religion, if security is rendered in terms of well-founded evidential beliefs.

The ambiguity in the use of the term "science" has arisen as a consequence of the failure to distinguish between science as "reflective enlightenment" and science as "content enlightenment." Science enlarges the scope of intellectual freedom to the extent that it provides the conceptual tools for liberating the mind from the tyranny of rigid and inflexible doctrine. Much of the confusion about the status and value of science within medicine derives from a collapsing of the above distinction, transforming the content of science, including its methodology, into the criterion of its enlightenment. Where science was once a force against authoritarianism, helping to break the spell of oppressive religious dogma, it has come ironically to cast an authoritarian spell of its own in the form of scientism. While religious salvation was once the prerogative of the institutional church, intellectual salvation has become the prerogative of the scientific establishment.

Our contention is that insofar as reductionist science has come to define the orientation of conventional medicine, not only the content but the methodology of conventional medicine have ceased to be imaginatively subversive. Medical scientism has lost its power to challenge inherited medical belief, because it is the bioreductionist disposition in medicine that itself now constitutes the inheritance. Reductionist science has, as part of its natural epistemic evolution, questioned, modified, and revised certain of its doctrines, but the questioning has almost invariably been set within a framework of reductionist methodology which is not itself questioned. This is true even in the case of conceptual revolutions, since paradigm shift is movement from one kind of science to another, not movement from science to a perspective which itself challenges movement in scientific terms. The challenge reductionist science presents to itself in respect of its content is not the salutary challenge heretical science formerly presented to religion. The institutionalization of reductionist medical science has deprived medical science of the power to call itself in question.

One need only consider the traditional character of health education to determine the extent to which science is embedded in and conditions learning. It is ironic that in schools the "facts" of health science are taught in as dogmatic a manner as were the "facts" of religion. What health science is thought to offer is a body of knowledge, to be learned, and expanded upon. The medical scientist has replaced the high priest, but there has been no relinquishment of the power and authority attached to the office. The state-sanctioned school support for reductionist science has been sustained within medicine by vested interests much in the same way as dogmatic religion was sustained in earlier centuries by vested interests within the State. The myths are different but the philosophic disposition is the same. The more powerful the scientific establishment has become, the more oppressive has become the authority by which it is articulated. The richer it has become, the more it has had to lose from those conceptual challenges that would deprive it of some of its wealth. It is urged by Stalker and Glymour that there is no knowledge outside of science, yet as we have tried to show earlier we do not have even a tolerably coherent epistemic account of what it means to say that we have knowledge within it.

Medical education in particular, for example, has never been more "authority-ridden" and conformist than it is now, though the form of authority in the guise of scientific methodology has perhaps become more subtle. More is done, that is to say, to create the impression that we nurture the critical faculties, and to encourage the suggestion that medical students really are "thinking for themselves." The rub is that the context of reflection is so rigidly circumscribed by what is deemed to be the objective and rational method of reductionist science that the exercise is little more than an idle ritual. Wholistic heretics within medicine, not unlike earlier scientific heretics within religion, suffer considerable hardships, not to be underestimated.

Summary

We have in this chapter argued that the standard objections to wholistic medicine derive from a framework of interpretation which is itself epistemically suspect. Scientism, not open-minded intellectual enquiry, sustains the methodology of conventional medicine. Bioreductionism, we observed, is one rational approach to medicine, but not the only rational approach. To challenge the rationality of wholistic medicine on the ground that it does not admit of test misses the point that not even reductionist science can satisfy the canons of empiricist rationality if they are systematically applied. One cannot reject wholism as irrational merely because certain of its claims defy evidential assessment without impugning the rationality of the scientific enterprise, since science itself contains certain propositions which are also resistant to experimental test.

Defending the philosophy of medical wholism against charges of irrationality is one thing, to establish its claim to rationality quite another. The latter task requires the articulation of an integrated epistemic framework of wholistic medicine, and we admitted that to date no satisfactory account had been given. In an attempt to add to remedy this deficiency we will next consider the relevance of certain recent developments in the philosophy of science as they bear upon the foundations of health education.

CHAPTER 8

The quantum connection: Consciousness and the new paradigm of health education

Having attempted to establish that the critique of medical wholism launched by Stalker and Glymour derives from a philosophical position which is itself untenable, it should now be easier to appreciate the connections between medical wholism and the quantum domain to which wholists often allude. Let us now turn to this task.

We have seen that medical scientism embodies the view that the world and the human organism resemble a machine, analyzable into separate parts whose interrelations are governed by specific laws which admit of precise mathematical formulation. On the reductio-mechanist view physical reality is in essence *fragmented*, and discovering its true character depends upon reducing it to the material particles of which it is composed. The objective of classical physics of course is not limited solely to the analysis of the parts of the machine; its aim is to show also how the parts work together, thereby exhibiting patterns of organization in seemingly distinct tracts of experience which, when taken in conjunction, ultimately determine the character of experience as a whole.

With the advent of quantum physics has come a crystallized perception of a new and fundamentally different order in nature. According to this new perception nature does not yield its deepest secrets by being whittled down into smaller and smaller components in the reductionist hope of reaching absolutely simple building blocks of which everything else is made and can be understood. The paradox is that in the last analysis the purportedly primitive components in the reduction turn out to be so inextricable related that their coherent description depends upon the postulation of a world of seamless unity and indivisible wholeness. The ontology of primitive particles in expressed, that is to say, by way of their correlations with other particles. Subatomic particles exist relationally; the separateness and independence of their particulate reality are illusory and incompatible with the quantum theory by way of which they are defined.

Bell's theorem

Although there have been several developments in the history of quantum physics which attest to the fundamental indivisibility and systemic character of nature as a whole, none is perhaps more persuasive than Bell's theorem, first published in 1964. [1] The force of Bell's theorem is best apprehended as a development in the tradition of the Einstein-Podolsky-Rosen thought experiment, often referred to as the "EPR effect." The design of the experiment was motivated by Einstein's discomfort with Bohr's indeterministic interpretation of quantum physics. The debate centered on Einstein's unwillingness to accept Bohr's contention that the behavior of any specific quantum phenomenon depended upon the logic of its interconnections with the whole of quantum reality. To accept Bohr's view was tantamount to conceding a seemingly ineradicable indeterminacy at the quantum level, for how could a definitive causal account be given of events which are causally influenced by all other events? Without the possibility of identifying a specific casual sequence to explain, say, the transitional jump of an electron from one orbit to another, only a probabilistic or statistical account of causality could be given to accommodate the peculiar nature of quantum phenomena. In short, Bohr's interpretation required the rejection of the very concept of local causality and determinacy upon which classical mechanics had been built.

Moreover, to admit that quantum events were determined by the dynamics of the whole system of quantum phenomena, and not by local connections which were themselves governed by precise laws legislating the behavior of objects separated in space, was to challenge Einstein's view that the signal connections between such objects were proscribed by the speed of light. Rather than accept this conclusion, Einstein insisted that indeterminacy at the quantum level was merely a matter of not having all the facts: a matter, that is to say, of the existence of hidden variables still awaiting discovery. Bohr, too accepted that the theory of hidden variables would feature prominently within the quantum domain; the difference of view was that for Einstein the only hidden variables were those deriving from local causes. The EPR experiment can thus be reckoned as a bold attempt to demonstrate that Bohr's postulation of nonlocal causal explanations for quantum phenomena would require that superluminary communication was possible, a description which Einstein held to be a contradiction in terms. Using essentially the same experiment, it has taken the mathematical genius of Bell, nearly three decades later, to show that Einstein appears to have been mistaken on this point.

Although Bell's theorem is a highly technical mathematical construct, its implications for quantum physics can be distilled. What Bell's theorem provides is a coherent mathematical explication by way of which to define the instantaneous-measurement effect between twin particles separated in space. Consistent with Bohr's interpretation of quantum reality, Bell's theorem demonstrated a fundamental connectivity among what have traditionally been regarded in classical mechanics as separate and logically autonomous parts of the universe. There is a wholeness to the universe, on this view, which defies reduction to independent and isolated material components. Appreciation of this wholeness requires that we reconceive the basic categories of scientific interpretation. On the classical view, the world could be understood by reducing its complex constituents to their fundamental parts and then determining the relations among the parts. The properties of the parts and the nature of their interconnections were thought to be sufficient to determine the logical character of the whole.

What Bell's theorem tells us mathematically represents a radical departure from this tradition. On the new view, it is the *whole*, the organizational pattern of the entire system, that is, which determines the patterns of its components and the properties and behavior of its parts. Bell's theorem thus signals a whole reconceptualization of the classical concept of a universe made up of separate bits whose relations admit of precise mathematical formulation in accord with the principle of local causes. At the deepest level of structure we have instead a universe of fundamentally interconnected elements whose specific character is itself a manifestation of the dynamics of interdependency which serves to express the unity of the entire system. The elements are not independent and isolated; they are in some almost mystical sense undifferentiated facets of an indivisible whole. Bell's theorem shows that material objects signify not individual things or entities, but patterns of probabilities expressing interconnections among the various presentations of a unified and systematic whole. This is why nonlocal causal connections do not correlate with signal communications in the conventional Einsteinian sense. Conventional signals such as the speed of light presuppose the very universe of independent, spatially separated objects which Bell's theorem impugns. [2] By radically reconceiving the structure of matter itself, quantum physics provides a coherent conceptual scheme in which instantaneous communication is possible without reference to the speed of light.

Bohm's implicate order and holograms

Concerned to elaborate the quantum concept of the universe as a cosmic web of interconnections, David Bohm has proposed an ingenious account of the nature of the interface between nonlocal connections and local connections.[3] Underpinning the probability relations which define the subject matter of quantum physics is a deeper or "nonmanifest" substratum which he calls the "implicate order." At this deeper level the structural interdependencies to which Bell's theorem alludes are not spatiotemporally constrained. To put it differently, the whole of quantum reality is somehow "enfolded" or in a special sense contained in each of its parts. The fundamental order of the universe is enfolded into the process of its instantiation. Its instantiation is the world of ordinary consciousness, what we generally see, hear, and experience, what Bohm calls the "explicate order," the events of which have traditionally been explicated by reference to the principle of local causes.

The analogy employed by Bohm to depict the quality of enfoldment is the hologram, inasmuch as the whole is deemed to be encoded in each of its parts. It was Dennis Gabor who in 1947 anticipated the principle of holography, a discovery which eventually brought him a Nobel Prize. It was not until the invention of the laser, however, that the initial construction of a holograph took place. Holograms involve a process akin to that of lensless photography in which light waves approximately the same frequency are passed through a half-silvered mirror. Light waves from a laser, being in general of the same frequency, are used for this purpose. The mirror directs some of the coherent light onto a photographic plate, reflecting other waves onto the object which is to be photographed. At the same time the object is situated in such a way that light will be deflected from the object onto the photographic plate, thereby colliding with the beam passing through the mirror. The resultant interference pattern is recorded as a hologram on the photographic plate.

If a laser beam is now passed through the photographic plate, a distinct three-dimensional image or picture of the object is projected so that it hangs eerily, suspended in space a short distance from the plate. This is in itself quiet remarkable, but even more remarkable is the fact that if light from a laser is used to illuminate any part of the resultant hologram, the pattern which emerges is simply a reconstruction of the whole hologram. Depending upon the size of the piece of the hologram illuminated, the resultant image will be more or less detailed and clear, though to be as sharply defined as the original object, it would be necessary to have a photographic plate of infinite extension. No matter how small the selected portion of the original hologram, it contains some information about every part of the illuminated object. The whole of the object is thus somehow encoded in each of its parts. It is in this sense that Bohm proposes that the structure of the universe embodies principles akin to those which depict the sense of the hologram. Although our ordinary consciousness of the world may encourage a reductionist description of the whole by reference to the independently existing parts which constitute it, the deeper structure, as intimated in the foregoing analysis, reveals a seamless, indivisible unity in respect of which the whole universe is mysteriously enfolded in each of its parts. Bohm's emphasis, however, is not so much on the structure of objects as with the structure of the dynamical movement or rhythm of the universe, a movement out of which all "objective" representations flow. Bohm introduces the term "holomovement" to express the dynamics of the enfolded ground or implicate order which sustains the world of "manifest entities" as we know them in commonsense terms. Even space and time are enfolded in the holomovement, as is consciousness itself. Indeed, the world of mind and the world of matter are for Bohm interdependent, and though not correlated by local causes, they are intimately connected by nonlocal ones, being projections of a mutual enfolding of an implicate order of the universe which transcends consciousness and matter, as we know them.

To relieve the obscurity of the concept of enfoldment and implicate order, Bohm uses the example of glycerin diffusion[4] The example is simple and effective. Imagine that we have two concentric cylinders, the smaller of which is placed inside the larger, while the space between them is filled with a clear viscous fluid such as glycerin. If we now deposit a droplet of insoluble ink onto the surface of the glycerin, a well defined black spot will remain intact. Suppose now that the larger cylinder is rotated in a clockwise direction. With the motion of the cylinder the ink will be drawn out into a thread-like form which becomes thinner and thinner until it eventually disappears altogether. Although the ink droplet is no longer part of the "explicate" or unfolded order of the system, it is still present in an implicate sense, having been enfolded into the glycerin. If the cylinder if now rotated in counterclockwise fashion, the droplet will gradually reconstitute itself, becoming progressively visible as the previously invisible thread darkens.

According to Bohm, order and unity are enfolded in the universe in much the same way that the ink droplet is enfolded in the glycerin. Considering the ink droplets as subatomic particles, it is clear that they may be discontiguous, separated by vast spatial distances, and yet be connected and interdependent in the implicate order. Similarly, if the universe is like a hologram with order and unity manifest throughout its total dynamics, then each part of the universe contains within it the organizational patterns of unity sufficient to reconstitute the unity of the whole. The form and dynamics of the implicate order are thus encoded within every part of the explicate order. In what would seem the endpoint or culmination in reductionist division, the elementary particle, whatever it may be, would seem to enshrine the fundamental unity and interdependency of the entire cosmos.

Gaia: the living earth

The time has now come, however, to distil from this cauldron of seemingly arcane ideas, some principles of relevance to the goal of education for health. Although the emergent philosophy of "wholistic science" which derives from the aforementioned developments has momentous implications for specific reforms within a number of different areas of education such as science education and environmental education, we will in what follows address ourselves to the adumbration of what we call an "Epistemic Wholism," as we believe that it provides an important key to the comprehensive philosophical framework within which reform in each of these areas can occur.

Our traditional theory of knowledge assumes a distinction between the knower and the known, between subject and object if you prefer. Within conventional science the aim has been to objectify our observations of nature by detaching ourselves from it. The world exists, so we have been led to believe, independently of what we say and think about it, or even of how we behave towards it. Realist epistemology rests firmly upon this presumption. Institutionalized distinctions between the subjective and objective domains of knowledge are – as we argued earlier – tenuous and we would now argue that the distinctions between subject and object, mind and matter are equally tenuous and misleading. In the light of the foregoing discussion of quantum interconnectivity, *consciousness* can no longer be described unambiguously as an element which admits of isolation and extraction from the external world. In the sense of Bohm's implicate order, consciousness is itself an essential feature of the underlying order and unity of the universe. The topology of nature cannot exclude the way in which consciousness is enfolded into it. Nature cannot be objectified in the required epistemic sense because in essence we have ourselves become an element in the subject matter we are trying to observe. We cannot separate ourselves from nature, because we are, in the radically wholistic interpretation of Bell's theorem, a part of it. In our attempts to measure and describe the world "outside ourselves," we now find that we are at one and the same time measuring and describing ourselves.

Another theoretical development which contributes to a new understanding of our basic bond to nature is the Gaia hypothesis. Given the bold affirmation of quantum interconnectedness and of the seamless unity of all things, it is possible to reconceptualize our relationship to nature in such a way that our oneness with it is justified by the epistemology upon which the affirmation of unity rests. The conventional view has been to mark a distinction between animate and inanimate matter between things that are living and things that are not. On the conventional view the earth is not a living thing. Within the tradition of science, however, the work Ilya Prigogine, to be discussed fully in the next chapter, has come to serve as a reminder that the distinction may not be as clear as one might suppose. "Dissipative chemical structures," as Prigogine refers to them, exhibit most of the dynamic features of self-organization characteristic of living systems, including primitive manifestations of "mental processes." Capra suggests that "the only reason why they are not considered alive is that they do not reproduce or form cells." [5]

Similarly, the boundaries thought to differentiate a living organism from its environment are not as uncontroversial as one might expect. Certain organisms may justifiably be considered dead in one environment and alive in another. Viruses, for example, are only partly self-sufficient and exist on the border between living and nonliving matter. Unable to multiply independently of the cellular context, their organizational dynamics appears to be nonfunctional outside cells.

Awareness of the intricate weave which patterns a dynamics of cosmic interconnectivity makes it easier to appreciate that the distinction between living and nonliving systems cannot be laid down unambiguously once and for all. It is out of this context of appreciation that the Gaia hypothesis has been resurrected, refined, and reconceptualized. Fashioned after a powerful ancient myth and named after Gaia the Greek goddess of the earth, the hypothesis has been interpreted by some as stating that Earth as a whole is a single living organism. Given that we normally approach systems microscopically, the Gaia hypothesis requires a shift of perspective whereby we view life through what has been called the "macroscope" of the Earth. Inasmuch as Earth, on this view, is a living system of which we are a part, it is difficult for us to detach ourselves from it in such a way that, having done so, we are disposed to regard it as living rather than nonliving.

The two main proponents of the Gaia hypothesis are James Lovelock, a chemist, and Lynn Margalis, a microbiologist. Lovelock says, "I have frequently used the word Gaia for the hypothesis itself, namely that the biosphere is a self-regulating entity with the capacity to keep our planet healthy by controlling the chemical and physical environment."[6] Depending upon how we regard nature, our place in it will be very different. We will see that if Gaia does exist, it follows that we and other living things can best be regarded as components in dynamic interrelation and partnership within the vast system of cosmic organization we know as the Earth. In support of the hypothesis of Gaia as a complex system in which the atmosphere, oceans, soil, and even the Earth's biosphere function collaboratively to ensure an optimal physical and chemical environment for life, Lovelock advanced an impressive argument deriving in large part from the Second Law of Thermodynamics and other laws of physical chemistry.

On the thermodynamic assumption that living systems take in, metabolize, and discard as waste, utilized energy and matter, Lovelock calculated that the presence of life, say, on a distant planet could be detected by its effects on its environment. On a planet devoid of life, for example, the chemical constituents of its surroundings (e.g., its oceans, atmosphere, soil, etc.) would settle into equilibrium at a rate roughly predicted by the laws of physical chemistry. When Lovelock applied his tests to the constituents of the Earth, he was astonished to find that, given the age of the Earth, the levels of chemical entropy differed in some cases by factors of millions from the levels predicted by the laws of physical chemistry. Particularly peculiar was the discovery that the levels of certain constituents such as those found in the atmosphere have remained relatively constant at levels conducive to the continuance of life on the planet. The actual concentration of oxygen in the air, for instance, is approximately [7] percent, the level optimal for life, though the predicted level is virtually zero. With just a slightly lower percentage of oxygen, survival would have become impossible for larger animals and flying insects.

Enumerating a number of such examples, Lovelock builds an impressive case to suggest that the entire planet is complicitous in a systemic manipulation of the chemical constituents requisite for life and health. He shows, for example, that despite past perturbations such as dramatic changes in atmospheric composition and significant elevations in heat radiation from the sun which would otherwise have critically disrupted life processes, the average temperature of most of the earth's surface has remained constant between 60 and 100 degrees Fahrenheit for literally hundreds of millions of years. It would also seem, he suggests, that the levels of oceanic salt are similarly regulated systematically in favor of the continuance of life. Present salt levels of the ocean, for example, are approximately 3.4 percent, of which about 90 percent is made up of the constituent ions of sodium chloride. Oceanic levels of salt have also remained constant for millions of years, despite the fact that salt is continually being swept into the oceans by rivers. Had the salt concentration of the oceans risen to 6 percent, most of the creatures of the sea would have perished as a consequence of the salt disintegration of their cell walls.[8]

The Gaia argument affirms that the Earth is a self-organizing, self-regulating, self-sustaining system, not unlike Prigogine's dissipative structures. While Lovelock is circumspect in his judgement that the Earth is a living organism, he has no hesitation in urging that its systemic nature is teleologically oriented towards the continuation of life. Although the total system can withstand and, indeed, may benefit from certain perturbations by being raised to a higher level of complexity, other perturbations such as nuclear pollution can overwhelm the feedback mechanisms in such a way that the integrity of the whole is in jeopardy. On this view the goal of health cannot be divorced from the goal of planetary balance. In the end, humanity is part of a larger living system whose organizational integrity depends in part upon the moral integrity and environmental consciousness of humanity. Let us consider this point further.

Away from a technology of aberration

The fundamental interdependency to which Bell's theorem alludes also inspires a profound paradigm shift in the covert value-orientation which underpins our traditional theory of knowledge. In our futile efforts to detach ourselves from nature to achieve a neutral perspective from which to view it, we inadvertently sever a relationship of basic bonding to nature which is integral to our viewing it wholistically. Rather than sensing our oneness with nature, we see ourselves as distinct from it and we are thus disposed to use the faculty of consciousness to gain control over it. The more detached and removed we become from nature, the easier it is to assume a posture of exploitation towards it. By way of the reductionist analysis of wholes into parts we effect a degradation of the integrity and identity of much of what we find in the natural world. Having reduced all living things to genetic complications of DNA, for example, we feel less contrite of heart in using genetic engineering to manipulate the impersonal building-blocks out of which all living things are made. There is less conscience and responsibility in manipulating the chemical substances of which human beings are composed than in manipulating human beings themselves. We have as a culture approached the Earth with the same exploitative tendency. We have robbed the environment of its identity through reductionist descriptions, thereby facilitating, in terms of moral responsibility, the prodigal manner in which we convert its resources into practical utilities for seemingly unlimited consumption.

It is easier to talk of uprooting trees than of uprooting forests or of disrupting ecosystems. Construing ourselves as separate from nature, we have been misled into thinking that nature is an adversary to be dominated, controlled, and subdued. Consistent with this approach, we have evolved a theory of knowledge which is tantamount to a theory of power over nature. Knowledge is expressed and implemented as power and control. The use of fire provides a good example of how knowledge, motivated by power, gives rise to a technology inspired by dominance. One crucial sociocultural difference between humankind and the animal world is that humankind has learned to use fire. Not only is it the case that animals neither make nor use fire, it is salutary to remind ourselves that they are instinctually frightened by it. Knowing how to make and use fire has thus given humankind a power over the animal world which is definitive of its dominance over all living things. Fire has also supplied the basis for a technology of dominance over the nonliving world of resources stored within Earth's bosom. Affording a technology for melting down the Earth's surface, fire has replaced the use of muscle power as the mechanism whereby the elements of the Earth are recast in "man's" own image.

Influenced and oriented by the sociocultural dominance of patriarchy, we have come to regard nature as a woman to be mastered and subdued. Although we will not at this late stage of the book pursue this divagation here, it is arguable that the metaphors by virtue of which we have described the world in patriarchal terms (e.g., "mother earth," "she blows a gale," etc.) are not accidental. At a deep level in the reaches of the human psyche, we characterize the Earth as a woman because the rape of the Earth and the rape of woman represent, in the collective unconscious, one and the same attitude of power and domination.[9]

The desire for mastery over the environment has led to the evolution of a marriage between knowledge and technology which seeks to maximize our expropriation of the Earth's resources while minimizing the time and effort devoted to the task. The biography of the growth of knowledge betrays and reiterates our insatiable appetite for power. The technology of fire, or what has come to be referred to as "pyrotechnology," culminates in the development of the ultimate symbol of fire power, the nuclear bomb. [10] With the development of the nuclear bomb we have shown ourselves capable of optimizing our power over the environment via a technology which neglects the extent to which the Earth is disempowered in consequence. The nuclear crisis we now face defies assessment as a historical aberration. It is the logical outcome of our hunger and thirst for power. We have sought total mastery and control over the physical world, and the exploitation of nature which has resulted from our traditional theory of knowledge has been consistent with that end. Unwittingly, we have perpetuated a theory of knowledge which, far from being neutral in respect of the subject matter of which it treats, promulgates the values of exploitation, domination, and control. The scientific establishment and its sundry social manifestations reflect the extent to which the theme of power has been sanctioned institutionally across our culture, not only in our educational system, but in our economic and political system, even down to the advertisements with which we are bombarded daily.

Towards wholistic epistemology of health education

Implicit in Bell's theorem and the subsequent developments in "wholistic science" which have followed from it are new principles of epistemic understanding, and the time has come to conclude by making these explicit. We have observed that our traditional theory of knowledge presupposes a universe made up of independent and isolated entities which in various combinations constitute the whole. Human consciousness is independent of the things of which it is conscious.

On Bohm's interpretation of quantum physics, and according to Bell's ingenious defence of it, the universe is one seamless and indivisible unity, the dynamics of which entail an intricate web of interdependencies and interconnections among its elements. Nor is Bell's theorem intended simply as a characterization of the subatomic domain. It is the character of the dynamics of the whole cosmic order which determines the property and behavior of its elementary constituents, as well as the complex events which take place within it. On this view human consciousness is not something logically distinct from matter, as our thoughts themselves impact upon matter and thus shape the world through a constellation of synchronicities of which science is only just becoming aware. The universe is a vast and complex dynamical system of which we are ourselves an integral component. We are, on this view, not separate from nature, but in partnership with it. A theory of knowledge oriented towards domination and power over the environment is therefore ineluctably self-defeating. "Epistemic Wholism," as we conceive it, is concerned not to disempower nature, but to empower it through partnership rather than colonization. Epistemic Wholism represents an approach to knowledge in which participation, not domination is the key factor. In place of power and control are empathy and connection. The aim is not to exploit human consciousness to achieve control but rather to achieve connection, relationship, and balance through consciousness. Knowing involves seeing the fundamental interrelationships which express the character of the whole. We must learn to discern how our participation in the dynamical process of indivisible unity represents an investment in the future rather than an extractive lien on the past.

An example of this participatory concept of knowledge can be seen in the contrast between conventional and what has been called "New Age Architecture." Traditionally, we have constructed our houses and buildings though they were fortresses against the onslaught of nature. Imperializing their environment, they expropriate massive quantities of energy to sustain their separateness from the world outside them. It has been noted for example, that the world's tallest building, the Sears Roebuck Tower in Chicago, requires more energy resources in one day than the neighboring city of Rockford, Illinois, whose population is approximately 150,000 people. [11] Guided by different considerations and a participatory epistemology, New Age architects seek a better understanding of how a building can be an environment within an environment. Seeking in what is constructed to extend the environment rather than to disrupt it, New Age Architecture is cognizant of the manner in which a design can capture the integrity and rhythm of an environment, incorporating the dynamics of the surrounding ecosystem to minimize the extractive features of the technology employed.

Whether the power of pyrotechnology has genuinely advanced our mastery over the environment is, we would suggest, a moot point. What seems clear is that the power of pyrotechnology and the theory of knowledge which has generated it, have – as Rifkin suggests – not served to make us more secure.[12] The unbridled logical extension of the quest for power and domination is tantamount to destruction and dissolution, degradation not only of the environment but of ourselves. The traditional theory of knowledge, and the valued orientation which undergirds it, has brought us to the brink of extinction. The only consolation is that we still have the power to choose how we define ourselves and our relationship to nature. The blinded giant of Science had led us to a new consciousness of the limitations of conventional science. The time has come to return the gift of sight to the blinded giant.

The wholistic approach to the epistemology of health is concerned to integrate into a coherent educative theory not only the psychological and biological aspects of illness and disease but the sociocultural and ecological manifestations which effect their nature and expression. In essence the biological and cultural dimensions of the aetiology of illness and disease cannot be separated. Social isolation, for example, may contribute as significantly to cancer as exposure to radiation. Similarly, the spiritual dimensions of health can be seen to play a much more important role in health than the bioreductionist tradition in medicine has been inclined either to suppose or to allow. The meaning of one's life, for example, or indeed whether one ascribes to it any meaning at all, will be seen to be of fundamental relevance to the wholistic understanding both of what it means to be ill and of what is necessary either to maintain good health or to be restored to it. To heal is in part to make whole, and to make whole is in part to heal.

Wholism in health represents a salutary redressing of the balance previously in favor of the bioreductionist model. The difficulty is, however, that wholism entails the integration of biological and sociocultural factors for which there is currently no coherent epistemic framework of accommodation. The move to wholism in medicine must be accompanied by the articulation of a different epistemic paradigm from that which underpins bioreductionism. Couched in the framework of reductionist epistemology, the rejection of bioreductionism as the dominant methodology of medicine is an idle ritual, for the conceptual tools required to sustain wholism are systematically denied by the epistemology that sustains reductionism. What is needed is a theory of knowledge sufficiently rich to incorporate both the empirical and meta-empirical dimensions of human understanding.

The momentum of Newtonian mechanics has carried reductionism far into the twentieth century despite what should otherwise have been the sobering influence of quantum physics. We have seen that on the quantum view the world does not admit of decomposition into absolutely fundamental constituents such as atoms or their parts which exist independently of other such constituents. The universe is rather a web of interconnections; objects at the atomic and subatomic level do not have an ontic identity separate from the way in which they relate to other objects. It is not so much that the universe is a machine without parts, as that its parts cannot be treated as the parts of a machine. Quantum objects and events, moreover, are not susceptible of a casual-mechanical description, for there is no logically independent thing of which there could be such a description. Every quantum event is ultimately influenced by every other event, including our attempts to record and monitor those influences. As Heisenberg pointed out, the whole concept of deterministic causality breaks down, since observation is by its very nature a disruption and a distortion of what we would wish to measure.[13] On the quantum view there is an order to the universe, but its logical character is relative and to be expressed statistically, in terms that is, of probabilities. The deeper the level of reality probed, the more probabilistic will become its description. The more fundamental the constituents, the more fundamental their interconnections and interrelations to what goes on elsewhere in the universe as a whole. Quantum theory has given rise to an account of the universe as a unified whole, constituted of complex sets of relationships whose specific description depended upon its relative place in the whole.

Epistemic Wholism reflects our concern to express epistemology in the context of a universe of fundamental interrelations. In this universe there are no ultimate constituents of matter to which all matter can be reduced, independently of their relations to other constituents. Accordingly, knowledge of the universe demands more than is afforded by a reductionist epistemology which uses analysis to decompose knowledge into its ultimate and unchanging foundations. There are foundations of knowledge whose logical constituents are epistemic primitives, but epistemic primitives are neither ultimate nor changing. They simply provide the measure of our descriptions of ways of describing the whole. In this sense the fallibilist realism is a commitment to ontological pluralism. There may be a world which exists independently of what we say and think about it, but it is our 'sayings' and our 'thinkings' that constitute its epistemic subject-matter. Ontological pluralism is in essence tantamount to the admission that there are many such 'sayings' and 'thinkings,' and that we shape the world by what we say and think.[14]

Epistemic primitives thus belong less to the realm of what is described than to frameworks of description. We create and extend the world by describing it. Indeed, we sometimes forget that thought is itself reality, though not every thought is a depiction of reality. The difficulty is that, setting aside pallid examples of variant description whose compliance class admits of semantic transformations from the one to the other, we have no Archimedean framework for the transformation of the semantic descriptions of physics into the semantic descriptions of psychology, medicine, or even religion. Reductionism, as we have observed, will almost ineluctably force conformity at the expense of diversity. Epistemic Wholism, on the other hand, seeks to preserve diversity at the expense of conformity. The unity of knowledge at which it aims comes not from the comparisons of frames of semantic descriptions with some Archimedean world independent of description, for there is no world undescribed in virtue of which descriptions of it can be validated. Inasmuch as the world is not just out there awaiting discovery, the quest for knowledge must be reconceived as something more than the quest for truths about the world so conceived. The growth of knowledge depends not so much upon some independent reality underpinning our descriptions, as upon the systematic form of conceptual organization embracing them, and it is this which is the referent of comprehensive wholism.

The concept of reality unencumbered by description is displaced by the concept of "realities" which are versions of it, and the value of reduction, biological or otherwise, is proportional to the extent to which it contributes to the integration of parts into wholes. The effect of Epistemic Wholism is thus to counter fragmentation, and in so doing, to synthesize diversity where possible, and to explain the failure of synthesis, where not. To achieve this, Epistemic Wholism obliges the discernment of interconnections among frames of reference, projecting them into new constellations of meaning and understanding. Notice, however, that the growth of knowledge is not on this view coterminous in extension with the accumulation of truths. Despite this seemingly radical departure from the orthodox affirmation of the necessary connection between knowledge and truth, comprehensive wholism benefits from the heresy. In defense of this claim we are not compelled to sever the connection between knowledge and truth in its entirety, but only to show that the role played by truth in the growth of knowledge has been grossly exaggerated.

It is obvious that the domain of truth and the domain of knowledge are not coextensive. To suggest, for example, that the knowledge we currently possess exhausts the domain of truth would be decidedly presumptuous. The admission that there are some truths which are not known seems so uncontroversial as to make further discussion of it fatuous. Reflection upon the history of science also makes it clear that there is as much warrant for the claim that the growth of knowledge consists in the accumulation of falsehoods as in the accumulation of truths. After all, the asymmetry between truth and rationality has permitted a history of science in which even the most carefully reasoned beliefs have, despite their rational entitlement, led to a failure of truth. Another way of thus seeing the process is in terms of the movement from one set of falsehoods to another, not from one set of truths to another. As a result of incessant adjustments of truth-value across the system of science, there is now at least a certain reverence for the view that among the sentences to which we have on the best available grounds attributed truth are sentences in respect of which the attribution of truth is gratuitous. The foregoing points will no doubt be familiar, though the persistent inclination to identify the growth of knowledge with the accumulation of truths would suggest that the connection is more subtle than has often been supposed.

Part of the difficulty may arise from having conflated two quite separate logical relations. The first is what would appear to be the sacrosanct relation between knowledge and truth. This first relation is sustained by the orthodox and unchallenged dictum that one cannot know what is false. This is not the account against which we are here inveighing, though we are not convinced that its privileged position is altogether deserved. It is the second and rather different relation to which we are here addressing ourselves. It is the relation that exists between the growth of knowledge and the accumulation of truths. The comprehensive epistemic wholism we have espoused impugns this second relation rather than the first. One obvious reason for this discrimination is that Epistemic Wholism is concerned primarily with the integration, ordering, and interpretation of whole systems of propositions, not simply of the syntactic components of a system which are semantically replicated by its extension. Inasmuch as the medium for truth-conveyance is constructed propositionally, the relation between knowledge and truth predominates. On the view we are advancing here, attention is shifted from questions of propositional truth to a question of the growth of knowledge which is only partly dependent upon them. The medium for the growth of knowledge is not propositions, even true ones, but systems of beliefs and the representational exemplifications deriving from their combination on the one hand, and their integration with symbol-systems such as art, music, and poetry on the other hand. One major impetus for this shift of emphasis in respect of the former is the wholistic assumption that a comprehensive symbolic system yields more meaning than is entailed in the aggregation of the particular symbolic components of which it is composed. To put this in the idiom of a shibboleth, "the whole is greater than the sum of its parts." It is one thing to say this, of course: it is quite another to show it. Let us at least try.

In respect of a constellation of propositional beliefs, Epistemic Wholism requires that its propositional constituents be nontrivially conjoined. The aggregate of propositions satisfying this condition will be reckoned not simply as an enumeration of individual propositions P1, P2, and so on, but of their enumeration, along with the anatomization of the logical relations in virtue of which they cohere. Inasmuch as their particular relations generate differential consequences which cannot be derived from the separate conjuncts, the informativeness of the system as a whole is greater than the sum of its conjuncts, constructed independently of their interrelations.

It is the aim of Epistemic Wholism, however, to show that the growth of knowledge results not only from systems of propositions in integration, but from the interrelation of such systems with symbol systems such as music and art and perhaps religion, whose meanings do not admit of reduction to the propositional components which may from time to time partly express them. This is another reason why it would be better to render the concept of the "growth of knowledge" in terms of what might be called "cognitive insight" than with the traditional notion of the accumulation to truths. Cognitive insight captures the sense in which the symbolic frameworks of are or literature contribute categories of understanding capable of illuminating and extending the truth-carrying categories of cognitive belief systems. They achieve this not only by providing novel ways of perceiving their respective frameworks, but also by emphasizing or de-emphasizing the salience and priority of cognitive components of frameworks exogenous to their own symbolic organization. Cognitive insight reflects the incorporation into the search for knowledge of those elements of symbolic systems whose primary function is not in itself necessarily the production of literal truth. This will be so even in the case where the symbolic component is putatively propositional. Although some heuristic statements which serve to interrelate disparate systems in relevant logical propinquity might themselves be literally false, for example, they may nonetheless be "truth-generating." That some statements are literally false, of course, is not to say that they are devoid of metaphorical truth, and metaphorical truth can contribute as readily to cognitive insight as can literal truth. This is not to suggest that the primary role played in the advancement of cognitive understanding by, say, literature or art is to be assured by means of what literature or art exemplify in the form of either metaphorical or literal truth.

Truth, we have been urging, is not the only, or always the prime consideration in the growth of knowledge. Even where a truth-entitlement would seem to be warranted, we are helped little if the truths to which we are entitled are "trivial, irrelevant, unintelligible, or redundant; too broad, too narrow, too boring, too bizarre, too complicated. . . ."[15] Where the putative truths revealed by our investigation are to finicky, or do not fit harmoniously with other beliefs upon which our investigations are based, we may, as Goodman puts it, "choose the nearest amenable and illumination lie."[16] Having so chosen, we preserve the system which makes best sense of out total experience of the world, and it would be naïve to suppose that the system that does this best does so by virtue of its superior accumulation of truths. There is a multiplicity of ways in which truths can be organized, and their varying organization can reflect a multiplicity of truths. In either case the interpretation of the pattern of truth is something in addition to the truths which constitute the pattern.

It is the task of Epistemic Wholism to seek not just truth, but cognitive insight intuition, imagination, and creativity. Consistent with this goal, comprehensive Epistemic Wholism depends upon the recognition that the reductionist concept of truth is not the only clue to a deeper understanding of our world, or even of how best to effect the organization of our sundry versions of the truths of the world. Appreciation of this point is tantamount to the additional recognition that knowledge itself admits of description as a multifaceted concept. Indeed, it may be that neither knowledge nor truth is monolithic in logical structure. Cognitive progress, if it is to be achieved at all, must come from our willingness to interpret and unify the vast array of human experience, and to do so in such a way that our experience of the world is more comprehensive for the interpretation. The growth of knowledge lies in the evolution of wholistic consciousness, not the accumulation of reductionist truths.

Summary

To remedy the deficiency of an integrated epistemic framework of wholistic medicine we considered the relevance of certain recent developments in the philosophy of science as they bear upon the foundations of health education. From Bell's Theorem and Bohm's "implicate order" we tried to establish a philosophical ground for the fundamental interdependence of all things and events. Thus, all healing ultimately becomes self-healing, and all self-healing ultimately becomes cosmic healing. Examination of the Gaia hypothesis further reinforced the picture of the fundamental patterns of interrelation which govern the cosmos, and emphasized the importance of the role played by humankind in the overall systemic organization of ecological planetary health.

Consideration was then given to Epistemic Wholism as a comprehensive knowledge base from which to project the philosophical foundations of wholistic health. We saw that knowledge designed to achieve power and dominance foster a relationship with nature which, by virtue of its exploitive character, is inimical to health and in conflict with the Gaian approach to the environment. Health is not possible without a deep sociopolitical commitment to making the Earth a better place.

Finally, we turned our attention to the more tedious task of articulating the epistemological parameters of the philosophy of health. To argue for wholism in health requires more than extolling the virtues of wholism. Once emancipated from reductionist epistemology, we set ourselves the task of postulating a theory of knowledge sufficiently rigorous to replace it. In the end we urged that the correlate to wholism in health is a comprehensive wholism in epistemology, capable of sustaining the new research methodology which wholistic health would require. In proposing what we have dubbed "Epistemic Wholism," we have been concerned to impugn also the strongly entrenched belief in the nexus between the growth of knowledge and the accumulation of truths. If there is a truth in this, it comes in seeing that the two are not always one. Truth is not the only jewel in the crown of knowledge; cognitive insight is another hidden gem of enormous value.

Conclusion

Although a new paradigm for understanding the nature of reality is steadily emerging, a central argument of this book has been to show that its ramifications for the philosophy of medicine and health education have yet to be adequately articulated. We make no pretense that our present ratiocinations have adequately remedied the deficiency to which we allude, but it is to be hoped that the conceptual paths we have cleared will serve to make it easier for others inspired to push the frontiers of the field further ahead.

To achieve the goal of greater clarity and a deeper understanding of the problem, we commenced our journey with an exploration of the ancient origins of medicine, endeavouring from this point of departure to exhibit not just the historical development of medical science and practice, but of equal importance the epistemological perspectives enshrined within this development. With a determinate shift in the source of knowledge from religious 'revelation' to a belief in the reliability of our sensory faculties as the primary source of truth, the evolution of medical praxis took a major step in a new direction, as did the already evolving epistemology underpinning it. One outcome of sensory-based epistemology was the birth of 'mechanism'. Upon observation of the world it was judged that nature was less like a nurturing mother than like a working machine. This being so, the presumed best methodology for comprehending how the machine-like world worked and could be controlled, was by dissecting and breaking it down into the parts of which it was composed. The parts could then themselves be reorganized through determining the functional relationships between and amongst the parts. Since the source of knowledge was located in sensory experience, the inter-relationships of the parts were defined causally, as causal connectivity was believed to be the principle observable. This epistemological assumption in turn gave rise to the concept of the importance of empirical testability as the method of cataloguing truths about the world in categories and formulations that allowed them to be recast as scientific laws. The goal of such laws epistemologically speaking was the measure of predictability they gave to control the behavior of the machine-like things under investigation. The power to predict was then tied to the power of technology to regulate and consolidate the potential unfolding of the predictable behaviors of things or events. We have endeavoured to show that the conceptual connections between these various presumptions constituted an epistemology which in turn gave birth to the child of invention through the 'transformative subjugation' of nature. The methodology deriving from the epistemologies of power is thus reductionist on the one hand and mechanistic on the other, while Newtonian causal determinism is the ostensible goal of reductio-mechanistic intervention as a methodological quantifier.

Having set the theoretical context in terms of the reductio-mechanistic approach to science, the burden of the next section of the book was to show that the crisis in health confronting modern society is as much a philosophical problem as it is a technological one, entrenched in mechanist medical intervention. The scope and the limits of the crisis were teased out to expose the philosophical presumption of mechanist conceptions underpinning it. Appreciation of the limitations of conventional medicine and of the interweaving of epistemological dogmas into its practice made it easier for us to establish that the way forward would require a radical reconceptualization of the very foundations of medicine.

In place of a theory of knowledge driven by the preoccupation with power, dominance and control, we invited consideration of what Laura has elsewhere called the epistemology of empathy. The idea here was that instead of seeking to know the world as a way of dominating and controlling it, we can come to know the world by connecting with it via a modality of participatory consciousness processes that engender empathetic interaction with the whole of nature. It was argued that our need to control the world and thus to transform it into increasingly inert forms is inimical to advancing the goal of community health and integrated well-being. The need to control devices forms a need for power to conquer and dominate the things and people around us from which and from whom we feel separate. When we can see and feel both intellectually and emotionally by way of affective resonance, the seamless and indivisible unity of the world around us becomes clear. We also see that the path to integrated well-being is by way of the healing, a defining condition of empathetic connectivity and love. Nothing makes us weaker and sicker than hatred and fear, and nothing makes us stronger than wisdom, compassion and love.

The final section of the book develops the theory of participatory consciousness and empathetic epistemology within the context of quantum philosophy. The concept of the body is radically changed, as are the concepts of health and disease associated with it. Integrated well-being cannot be reduced to a treatise on physiological functionality and efficient bodily processes, though such matters are prerequisites to health. To heal is to make whole, and to make whole is to help people find a deep sense of purpose and passion sufficient to transcend the egocentric universe of fear, alienation and separation from the world in which we live.

Integrated well-being is a way of educating people not just to see the world through their eyes but to feel and connect with the world through their hearts. It is a way of feeling the world around oneself such that we come to recognise at the deepest level that we are not only what we eat - we are what we think. The truth in the end is that we embrace wellness by living purposively, passionately and empathetically in ways which allow us to feel our oneness with the world around us. Affective resonance is itself a form of consciousness that not unlike a magnet, draws the things that make us whole to us and us to the things that make us whole and well.

Notes / References

Introduction

1. R.S. Laura and A. Chapman (2007), "Philosophical Views on Educational Compuphilia", *Critical and Creative Thinking: The Australian Journal of Philosophy in Education*, 2007, vol. 15, No. 2.
2. C. Glymour and D. Stalker, "Engineers, Cranks, Physicians, Magicians," in D. Stalker and C. Glymour, (eds.), *Examining Wholistic Medicine*, 1985, Prometheus Books, New York, p. 27.
3. See, for example, M. Kaufman, *Homeopathy in America: The Rise and Fall of a Medical Heresy*, 1971, John Hopkins University Press, Baltimore, and H.Coulter, *Divided Legacy: The Conflict Between Homeopathy and the American Medical Association*, 1982, North Atlantic Books, Richmond, California.
4. See, for example, E. Erwin, "Wholistic Psychotherapies: What Works?" in Glymour and Stalker, *Ibid.*, p. 268.
5. L. Price, "Art, Science, Faith and Medicine: The Implications of the Placebo Effect," *Sociology of Health and Illness*, 1984, Vol. 6, No. 1, pp. 64-68.
6. *Ibid.*, p. 5.
7. C. Glymour, *Ibid*, p. 21.
8. J. S. Gordon, "The Paradigm of Wholistic Medicine," in A.C. Hastings, J. Fadiman, and J. S. Gordon, (eds)., *Health For The Whole Person*, 1980, Westview Press, Boulder, Colorado, pp. 8-9. See also J. S. Gordon and J. Fadiman, "Toward and Integral Medicine," in J. S. Gordon, D. T. Jaffe, and D. E. Bresler, eds., *Mind, Body and Health*, 1984, Human Sciences Press, New York, pp. 4-5.

Chapter 1: The epistemological evolution of reductionist medical science

1. See, for example, J. H. Warner, *Science in Medicine*, 1985 *Osiris*, 2d series, vol. 1, pp. 37-58.
2. C. Singer and E. A. Underwood, *A Short History of Medicine*, 1962, 2d ed., Oxford University Press, London, p. 1.
3. See also, V. Nutton, *Ancient Medicine,* 2005, Routledge, Oxon, pp 37-39.
4. *Ibid.,* p. 31.
5. C. Singer and E. A. Underwood, *A Short History of Medicine*, 1962, 2d ed., Oxford University Press, London, pp. 2-3.
6. See also, R. Porter, *Cambridge Illustrated History of Medicine*, 1996, Cambridge University Press.

7. See, for example, L. Feuerbach, "God as a Projection of the Human Mind," in J. Hick, (ed.), *Arguments for the Existence of God*, 1964, Macmillan, New York, pp. 191-203, and J. H. Beattie, "On Understanding Ritual," in B. R. Wilson, (ed.), *Rationality*, 1970, Basil Blackwell, Oxford, pp. 240-68.
8. See also, M. S. Micozzi, "Traditional Medicine Systems", in *Fundamentals of Complementary and Integrative Medicine,* 2006, Saunders Elsevier, p. 373.
9. See E. D. Pellegrino and D. C. Thomasma, *Philosophical Basis of Medical Practice*, 1981, Oxford University Press, Oxford, particularly their chapter "Critique of Medicine," pp. 82-99.
10. B. Inglis, *Natural Medicine*, 1980, Fontana, Glasgow, pp. 14-18.
11. See also, Australian Institute of Health Sciences, *Naturopathic Philosophy*, 2007, Australian Institute of Health Sciences, Canberra.
12. C .Singer, *ibid.*, pp. 143-44.
13. M. Micozzi, *ibid.,* pp. 54-55.
14. G. A. Doran, *Science Education in Medicine: An Application of Paul Feyerabend's Philosophy*, 1982. Unpublished Doctoral Thesis, University of Newcastle, Australia, p. 11.
15. See also, V. Nutton, *Ancient Medicine*, 2005, Routledge, Oxon, p. 31.
16. *Ibid.*, p.113.
17. See also, P. Strathern, *Medicine from Hippocrates to Gene Therapy*, 2005, Constable & Robinson, London.
18. A. Castiglioni, *A History of Medicine*, trans. E. B. Krumbhar, 1941, A A Knopf, New York, pp. 37-63.
19. C. Singer, *ibid.*, pp. 18-19.
20. A. Castiglioni, *op. cit.*, pp. 120-29.
21. See also, V. Nutton, *ibid.*, pp. 92.
22. H. E. Sigerist, *A History of Medicine*, 1955, Oxford University Press, Oxford, vol. 1, pp. 335-36. See also C. Singer, *op. cit.*, pp. 32-41.
23. See also, V. Nutton, *ibid.*, pp 72-87.
24. A. Castiglioni, *ibid.*, pp. 179-88.
25. See also, P. Strathern , *ibid.*
26. A. Castiglioni, *ibid.*, pp. 189-204. See also C. Singer, *,ibid.*, pp.51-59.
27. P. Strathern , *ibid.*
28. C. Singer, *ibid*, p. 59.
29. A. Castiglioni, *ibid*, pp. 217-26.
30. P. Strathern, *ibid*, p. 31.
31. A. Castiglioni, *ibid*, pp. 242-57.
32. C. Singer, *ibid*, pp. 67-76.
33. G. Venzmer, *Five Thousand Years of Medicine*, trans. M Koenig, 1972, Macdonald Press, London, pp. 100-107.
34. See also, R. Porter, 1996,"What is Disease", 1996, in *Cambridge Illustrated of History Medicine*, Cambridge University Press, pp. 82-118.
35. A. Castiglioni, *ibid*, pp. 258-64; see also C Singer, *ibid.*, p. 116.

36. P. Strathern , *ibid.*, pp. 59-61.
37. A. Castiglioni, *ibid.*, pp. 271-73.
38. G. Venzmer, *ibid.*, p. 109.
39. A. Castiglioni, *ibid.*, pp. 299-322; see also C Singer, *ibid.*, p. 73; see slso G Venzmer, *ibid.*, p. 113.
40. A. Castiglioni, *ibid.*, p. 338.
41. C. Singer, *ibid.*, pp. 81-83.
42. A. Castiglioni, *ibid.*, pp. 408-32.
43. P. Strathern, *ibid.*, pp 90-106.
44. A. Castiglioni, *ibid.*, p. 445.
45. P. Strathern, *ibid.*, pp.72-85.
46. C. Singer, *ibid.*, pp. 111-15.
47. R. Porter, *ibid.*, pp. 161-165.
48. F. Capra, *The Turning Point*, 1982, Fontana, London, pp. 267-68.
49. C Singer, *ibid.*, p. 116.
50. F Bacon, *Advancement of Learning and New Atlantis*, 1962, Oxford University Press, Oxford, p. 123.
51. *Ibid.*, p. 124.
52. R Descartes, *Treatise of Man*, 1972, Harvard University Press, Cambridge, pp. xxxi.
53. F Capra, *op. cit.*, p. 45.
54. C Singer, *ibid.*, pp. 132-138.
55. P Strathern P, *ibid.*, p. 129.
56. A Castiglioni, *ibid.*, pp. 522-524.
57. *Ibid.*, p. 519-521.
58. C Singer, *ibid.*, p. 200.
59. *Ibid.*, p. 169.
60. P Strathern, *ibid.*, pp. 163-167.
61. A Castiglioni, *ibid.*, pp. 609-12.
62. P Strathern, *ibid.*, pp. 156-163.
63. A Castiglioni, *ibid.*, p. 649.
64. *Ibid.*, p. 942.
65. *Ibid.*, pp. 712-24.
66. C. Singer, *ibid.*, pp. 200-202.
67. See also, Australian Vaccination Network, *Vaccination Roulette: Experiences, risks and alternatives*,1998, Australian Vaccination Network, Bangalow, Australia.
68. C. Singer, *ibid.*, p. 327.
69. A. Castiglioni, *ibid.*, pp. 672-73.
70. *Ibid.*, pp. 695-98.
71. P. Strathern, *ibid.*, pp 210-214.
72. A. Castiglioni, *ibid.*, p. 679.
73. *Ibid.*, p. 677.
74. *Ibid.*, pp. 805-11.
75. See also, Australian Institute of Health Sciences, *Naturopathic Philosophy,* 2007, Australian Institute of Health Sciences, Canberra.

76. See also, Australian Vaccination Network, *Vaccination Roulette: Experiences, risks and alternatives*, 1998, Australian Vaccination Network, Bangalow, Australia.
77. C. Singer, *ibid.*, pp. 379-80.
78. See also, Australian Institute of Health Sciences, *ibid.*
79. P. Strathern, *ibid.*, pp 300-306.
80. See also: R. Porter, *ibid.*, pp.184-185.
81. A. Castiglioni, *ibid.*, p. 813.
82. P. Strathern, *ibid.*, pp 328-333.
83. C. Singer, *ibid.*, p. 695.
84. *Ibid.*, p. 696.
85. A. Castiglioni, *ibid.*, pp. 682-83.
86. F. Capra, *ibid.*, p. 98.
87. C. Singer, *ibid.*, p. 658.
88. *Ibid.*, p. 507.
89. *Ibid.*, p. 507.
90. *Ibid.*, p. 505; see also A. Castiglioni, *ibid.*, p. 635.
91. *Ibid.*, p. 511.
92. A. Castiglioni, *ibid.*, p. 799.
93. *Ibid.*, p. 715.
94. *Ibid.*, p. 890.
95. *Ibid.*, p. 747.
96. C. Singer, *ibid.*, pp. 613-618.
97. E. Yoxen, *The Gene Business*, 1983, Oxford University Press, New York, pp. 62-64.
98. E. Yoxen, *ibid*, p. 103.
99. P. Strathern, *ibid.*, pp 394-395.

100.J. D. Watson and F. Crick, "Molecular Structure of Nucleic Acids," *Nature*, 1953, April 25.

101.P. Strathern, *ibid.*, pp 385-391.

102. J. D. Watson, *The Double Helix*, 1969, Mentor Books, New York, pp. 126-36.
103. T. Howard and J. Rifkin, *Who Should Play God?* 1977, Dell Publishing, New York, p. 24; see also H. Curtis, *Biology*, 1983, 4th ed., Worth Publishing, New York, p. 302.
104. H. Curtis, *ibid.*, p. 304.
105. E. Yoxen, *ibid.*, pp. 73-78.
106. P. Abbey, *Going Organic*, 2002, Allen & Unwin, Australia.
107. B. Gretchen and S. Druckery, *Culture on the Brink: Ideologies and Technologies*, 1004, Bay Press, Seattle.
108. M. Bremner, *Genetic Engineering and You*,1999, Harper Collins, London, p. 205.
109. M.. Frankel, "Genetic Engineering Should Not be Used to Improve Human Beings" in S Barbour *Genetic Engineering*, 2002, Thomson Gale, p. 27.
110. S. Barbour, *Genetic Engineering*, 2006, Thomson Gale, pp 9-14.

111. J. Rifkin, *Declaration of a Heretic*, 1985, Routledge & Kegan Paul, Boston, pp. 51-54.

Chapter 2 Scientism and the catastrophe of the modern health system

1. See, for example, R. Horne, *The Health Revolution*, 1985, Southwood Press, Marrickville, Australia, pp. 10-11; see also J. S. Gordon and J. Fadiman, "Towards An Integral Theory of Medicine", *ibid.*, p. 3.
2. P. Day, *Health Wars,* 2003, Credence Publications, Tonbridge, England, pp 21-30.
3. J. Robbins, *Healthy At 100,* 2006, Random House, Canada.
4. See, I. Illich, *Limits to Medicine*, 1976, Penguin Books, Harmandsworth, pp. 23-30; see also T. McKeown, *The Role of Medicine*, 1979, Princeton University Press, Princeton, pp. 29-44.
5. See also G.L.Armstrong, L.A. Conn , R. W. Pinner, "Trends in Infectious Disease Mortality in the United States During the 20th Century", 1999, *Journal of the American Medical Association*, 281, pp 61-66.
6. R. Horne, *ibid.*, p.10.
7. J.S. Gordon & J. Fadiman, *ibid.,* p.8
8. E. Hillary, "Big Medicine: The Sickness Industry" in E Hillary *Health Betrayal: Staying away from the Sickness Industry,* 1999, Synergy Books Pty Ltd, pp 60-77.
9. P.Day, ibid., p.27.
10. M. Ezzati, A. Friedman, S. Kulkarni & C. Murray,"The Reversal of Fortunes: Trends in County Mortality and Cross-County Mortality Disparities in the United States", 2008, *PLOS Medicine*, p. 66.
11. R. Taylor, *Medicine Out of Control*, 1979, Sun Books, Melbourne, p. 21.
12. *Ibid.*, p.21.
13. P.Day, ibid., pp 8-9.
14. Cancer Research United Kingdom, "Worldwide Cancers", Cancer Research UK, cited March 2008, http://info.cancerresearchuk.org/cancerstats/.
15. M. Gray, "The Leading Cause of Cancer Death in Women", *The Internet Journal of Academic Physician Assistance*, cited August 2008.
16. Cancer Research United Kingdom, ibid.
17. I. Hajjar & T. Kotchen, "Trends in prevalence, awareness and treatment of Hypertension in United States: 1988-2000", 2003, *Journal of the American Medical Association*, pp 199-206.
18. A. Scher, R. Lipton & W. Stewart, "Risk Factors for Chronic Daily Headache",2007, *Current Pain & Headache Reports*, pp 486-491.
19. E. Finkelstein, I. Fiebelkorn & G. Wang "National Medical Spending Attributable to Overweight and Obesity: How much and who's paying?", 2003, *Health Affairs*, pp 219-226.

20. D. Satcher, *Mental Health: A Report of the Surgeon General,* 1999, National Public Health Service, cited February 2008.
21. See "Aspirin", Internet Information Centre for Substance Related Risk Reduction, cited July 2008, www.drugtext.org.
22. NCD Health , "The Top 200 Prescriptions for 2003 in the United States", 2005 A Healthcare Information Company, cited August 2008.
23. J.S. Gordon & J. Fadiman, *ibid.*, p.5.
24. R. S. Laura, *Philosophical Foundations of Health Education*, 1990, Routledge, p.53.
25. M. Boudrealt, L. Fingerhut, *Injury Data and Resources for School Aged Children,* United States Department of Health and Human Services, 2004, United States Centre for Disease Control, cited July 2008 www.cdc.gov/nchs/ppt/duc2004/Boudreault_Fingerhut.ppt.
26. R. S. Laura, *ibid.*, p.53.
27. P. Bruckenwell, D. Jackson, M. Luck, J. Wallace & J. Watts, *The Crisis in Men's Health,* 1995, Community Health, United Kingdom, Bath.
28. F Capra, *ibid.*, p. 266.
29. M. Story & S. French S, "Food Advertising and Marketing directed at Children and Adolescents in the United States", 2004, *International Journal of Behaviour and Nutrition and Physical Activity.*
30. *Ibid.*
31. A. Gallo, "Food advertising in the United States: Americans eating habits, changes and consequences", in JM Harris, P Kaufman, S Martinez and C Price, *The United States Food Market System,* 1999, USDA 2002, cited August 2008, www.ers.usda.gov/publications/aer811.
32. Finkelstein, Fiebelkorn & Wang, *ibid.*, pp 219-226.
33. Laura, *ibid.,* p.53.
34. *P. Goygen, 2003.*
35. F. Capra, *ibid.,* pp 249-250.
36. *Ibid,*. p.248.
37. S. Cox, *US: Toxic Teflon: Compounds from Household Products found in Human Blood*, 2007, CorpWatch, cited March 2008, http://www.corpwatch.org/article.php?id=14295
38. NSWMA, *Hazardous Waste: Facts on File*, 2002, National Solid Waste Management Association, cited June 2008.
39. T. McKeown, *ibid.*, see particularly his ch. 13, "Dream, Mirage, or Nemesis," pp 176-89.
40. H. Benson, *Beyond the Relaxation Response*, with W. Proctor, 1985, Berkley Books, New York, p. 17.
41. I. Illich, *ibid.*, see particularly his ch. I, "The Epidemics of Modern Medicine," pp 21-44
42. *Ibid.*, pp 47-129.
43. F. Capra, *ibid.*, p. 7.
44. J Gordon and J Fadiman, pp 4-5; see also E .M Goldwag, *ibid.*, p. 10.

45. M. Leavitt, J. Gerberding & E. Sondik, *Health, United States: 2007,*2007, United States Department of Health and Human Services, Centre for Disease Control and Prevention & National Centre for Disease Statistics. See also J. Poisal, C. Truffer, S. Smith, A. Siskoic, C. Cowan & S. Keehan, "Health Spending Projections through 2016: Modest Changes Obscure Part D's Impact", in George Beller "The Rising Cost of Health Care in the United States: Is it making the United States globally noncompetitive", *Journal of Nuclear Cardiology*, vol. 15, no. 4, 2008.
46. *U.S. House of Representatives, Committee on Interstate and Foreign Commerce*, "Surgical Performance: Necessity and Quality," 1978, United States Government Printing Office, Washington D.C., pp 24-28.
47. *Ibid*., pp. 36-38.
48. G. Null, C. Dean, M. Feldman, D. Rasio & D. Smith, *Death By Medicine,* 2003, cited March 2008, http://koray.asklepion.org/DeathByMedicine.pdf.
49. R. Kuttner, "Market Based Failure: A Second Opinion on U.S. Health Care Costs", *Journal of New England Medicine*, 2008, no. 358, pp 549-551.
50. The Henry J. Kaiser Foundation 2007, *Employee Health Benefits 2007 Annual Survey*, cited July 2008 www.kff.org/insurance/7672/index.cfm
51. Centre for Disease Control, *Quick Facts: Economic and Health Burden of Chronic Disease,* 2008, cited March 2008 http://www.cdc.gov/nccdphp/press/index.htm#3
52. R. Dubos, *The Mirage of Health*, 1959, Harper & Row, New York, p.89.
53. See, for example, I Illich, *ibid*., pp. 26-29.
54. R. Porter, "The Contribution of the Biological and Medical Sciences to Human Welfare," *Presidential Address to the British Association for the Advancement of Science*, Swansea Meeting, 1971 (London: The Association, 1972) p. 95.
55. *Ibid*., pp 36-37.
56. Illich, *ibid*., p.35.
57. G. Null, *ibid.*
58. Centre for Drug Education and Research, Preventable Adverse Drug reactions: A Focus on Drug Interactions, cited March 2008, www.FDA.gov/CDER
59. *G. Null, ibid.*
60. R. S. Mendelsohn, *ibid*., p. 56.
61. P. Day, *ibid., pp 21-30.*
62. G. Null, *ibid.*
63. *Ibid.*
64. *Ibid.*
65. D. W. Bates, D. Cullen, N. Laird et.al, "The Nature of adverse events in hospitalized patients: results from the Harvard Medical Practice Study II", *Journal American Medical Association,* 1995, no. 324, pp 377-384.

66. Mendlesohn, *ibid., p.54.*
67. Illich, *op, cit., pp 37-40.*
68. G. Null, *ibid.*
69. See, for example, *U.S. House of Representatives, Committee on Interstate and Foreign Commerce*, "An Overview of Medical Malpractice," 94th Congress, 1st Session, 17 March 1975.
70. G. Null, *ibid.*
71. G. Null, *ibid.*
72. A. B. Bergman & J. S. Stamm, "The Morbidity of Cardiac Nondisease in School Children," *New England Journal of Medicine*, vol. 276, 1967, pp. 1008-13.
73. R. Taylor, *op. cit.*, pp. 51-53.
74. See also D. Jackson & R Soothill, *Is the Medicine Making You Il*l, Angus & Robertson: Sydney: pp 4-5.
75. D. Jackson & R. Soothill, *ibid., pp* 4-5.
76. *Ibid.*, pp 4-5.
77. *Ibid.*, pp 4-5.
78. *Ibid.*, pp 4-5.
79. R. Taylor, *ibid.,* p.53.
80. R. S. Mendlesohn, *op. cit.*, pp 57-58.
81. *Ibid.*, pp 61-63.
82. J. Piccinino & W. Masher, "Trends in contraceptive use in the United States: 1982-1995",1995, *Family Planning Perspectives*, pp 4-10.
83. Medelsohn, *ibid.*, p. 63.
84. *Ibid.*, p.65.
85. P. Day, *ibid.*, pp 70-73.
86. P. Day, *ibid.*, pp 70-73.
87. Mendelsohn, *ibid.*, pp 66-67.
88. R. Taylor, *op.cit.*, pp 63-64.
89. J. Lanman et. al., "Retrolental Fibroplasia and Oxygen Therapy," *Journal of the American Medical Association*, 1954, vol. 155, p. 223.
90. R. Taylor, *op. cit., pp 63-64.*
91. R. S. Mendelsohn, *op. cit.*, p.27.
92. *Ibid.*
93. *Ibid.*
94. R. Taylor, *op. cit.*, p.64.
95. S. Epstein, R. Bertell & B. Seaman B, "Dangers and Unreliability of Mammography: Breast Examination is a Safe, Effective and Practical Alternative", 2001, *International Journal of Health Services, no.* 31, pp 605-615.
96. S. Rice, *Some Doctors Make You Sick*, 1988, Angus and Robertson Publishing, North Ryde, Australia, p. 15.
97. Epstein, Bertell & Seaman, *ibid.*, pp 605-615.
98. R. Taylor, *op. cit.*, p. 64.

99. For a concise but accurate summary of the development of PNI, see S Locke and D Colligan, *The Healer Within*, 1986, E P Dutton, New York, pp. 19-24.
100. R. Taylor, *op. cit.,* p.64.
101.Cited from S. Locke & D. Colligan, *ibid.,* p.23.
102. *R. S. Mendelsohn, ibid., pp 22-23.*
103. Cited from S. Locke & D. Colligan, *ibid.,* p.23.
104. R. S. Mendelsohn, ibid., p.58.

Chapter 3 Taking our blinkers off: Tapping the potential for health through wholsim

1. D. Stalker and C.Glymour, *op. cit*., p. 10.
2. See also B.L. Beyerstein, *Alternative medicine and common errors of reasoning*, 2001, Acad. Med, vol. 76, pp. 230-237.
3. M. Saks, *Alternative therapies: are they wwholistic?,1997,* Complement Ther Nurs Midwifery, vol. 3, no. 1, pp.4-8.
4. *Ibid.*
5. *Ibid.*
6. L. McEvoy, A. Duffy, *Wholistic Practice- A Concept Analysis,* 2008, In Press, Nurse Educ in Pract.
7. J. Freeman, *Towards a Definition of Wholsim*, 2005, Br J Gen Pract, vol. 55, no. 511, pp. 154-155.
8. J. B. S. Haldane, *The Philosophy of a Biologist*, 1935, Clarendon Press, Oxford.
9. See also J. P. Carter, *Racketeering in Medicine: The Suppression of Alternatives*, 1992, Hampton Roads Publishing Company, Norfolk.
10. L. von Bertalanffy, *General Systems Theory*, 1972, Allen Lane, London.
11. Freeman, *ibid*., pp. 154-155.
12. R. Dubos, " Medicine Evolving," in D. S. Sobel, (ed), in *Ways of Health, ibid*., p. 23.
13. *Ibid*., p. 24.
14. See also J. Shackelford, *A Philosophical Path for Paracelsian Medicine*, 2004, Museum Tusculanum Press, University of Copenhagen.
15. For a more comprehensive account of this view see G. L. Engel, "The Nature of Disease and the Care of the Patient: the Challenge of Humanism and Science in Medicine," 1962, *Rhode Island Medical Journal*, vol. 45, pp. 245-51.
16. R. Dubos, "Medicine Evolving," *ibid*., p. 28.
17. D. Callahan, "The World Health Organisation Definition of Health," *Centre Studies*, 1973, vol. 1, New York, p. 78.
18. *Ibid*., p. 78.
19. See also, Health and Disease, cited August 2008, www.ucalgary.ca/~ereshefs/publications/Health%20and%20Disease.dc

20. Callhan, *Ibid., p.* 78.
21. *Ibid.*
22. H. Seigel, "To Your Health: Whatever That May Mean," *Nursing Forum*, 1973, vol. 12, p. 280.
23. M. Blaxter, Health, 2004, Polity Press, Cambridge.
24. See also C. Louise, *The Systems Principles That Underlie Naturopathic Medicine-The Human Being As A Complex System*, 2007, International Editors Retreat, Stevenson, Washington, April 1-5, (Draft Paper).
25. E. Laszlo, *The Systems View of the World: A Wholistic Vision of our Time*, 1996, Hampton Press.
26. See, for example, F. Capra, *ibid.*, pp. 289-95.
27. *Ibid.*, p. 75.
28. A. Hróbjartsson, P.C. Gøtzsche, *Is the placebo powerless? An analysis of clinical trials comparing placebo with no treatment,* 2004, J Int Med, no. 256, pp. 91–100.
29. Louise, *ibid.*
30. *Ibid.*
31. F. Capra, *The Web of Life: A new scientific understanding of living systems,* 1996, Anchor Books, New York.
32. *Ibid.*
33. *Ibid.*
34. L. Dossey, *Space, Time and Medicine*, 1982, Shambhala, Boulder, Co., p. 74.
35. *Ibid.*, p. 75.
36. Louise, *ibid.*
37. G. L. Engel, *ibid.*, p. 248.
38. I. Prigogine, *From Being to Becoming*, 1980, Freeman, San Francisco.
39. S. E. Jorgensen, "Application of Wholistic thermodynamic indicators", *Ecological Indicators*, 2006 vol., 6, no. 1, pp. 24-29.
40. M. Ferguson, *The Acquarian Conspiracy*, 1980, J. P. Tarcher, New York, p 165.
41. Jorgensen, *ibid.*
42. *Ibid.*
43. Cited from Lukas, "The World According to Ilya Prigogine," *Quest/80*, December 1980, p. 88
44. L. Dossey, *ibid.*, p. 83.
45. For further information on this point see A. Shaifee and M. Karimi, *On the Relationship between entropy and information*, 2008, cited June 2008, http://arxiv.org/ftp/quant ph/papers/0611/0611061.pdf
46. *Ibid.*
47. Jorgensen, *ibid.*
48. Capra, *ibid.*
49. *Ibid.*
50. M. Ferguson, *ibid.*, p. 166.
51. Louise, *ibid.*
52. L. Dossey, *ibid.*, p. 89.

53. H. Brody and D. S. Sobel, "A Systems View of Health and Disease," in D. S. Sobel, (ed)., *Ways of Health*, *op. cit.*, pp. 97-98.
54. L. Dossey, *ibid.*, pp. 90-91.
55. For a comprehensive examination of the role of stress in illness and disease, see H. G. Wolff, S. G. Wolff Jr., and C. C. Hare, (eds). *Life Stress and Bodily Disease*, 1950, Williams and Wilkins.
56. H. Weiner, *Frontiers of Stress Research*, 1986, based on a Symposium on "Stress," Palm Beach, Fl.; see also his *Psychobiology and Human Disease*, 1977, Elsevier, New York
57. M, S. Miccozi, *Fundamentals of Complementary and Integrative Medicine. 3rd ed.* 2006, St. Louis: Saunders Elsevier, St Louis.
58. C. N. Parkes, B. Benjamin, and R. G. Fitzgerald, "Broken Heart: A Statistical Study of Increased Mortality Among Widowers," *British Medical Journal*, 1969, vol. 1, pp. 740-43.
59. S. Locke and D. Colligan, *ibid.*, p. 71; they remind the reader also that forms of stress may be beneficial (Seyle labelled such stress factors as "*eustress*"), providing a challenge which some individuals thrive upon.
60. S.C. Segerstrom, S.E. Taylor, M.Kennedy, J.L.Fahey, "Optimisim is associated with mood, coping and immune change in response to stress", *Journal of Personality and Social Psychology*, 1998, vol. 74, no. 6, pp. 1646-1655.
61. M Ferguson, *ibid.*, p. 253.
62. J. Denollet, N. Stroobant, H. Rombouts, T.C. Gillebert & D.L. Burtsaert DL, *Personality as independent predictor of long term mortality in patients with coronary heart disease*,1996, cited October 2007, http://arno.uvt.nl/show.cgi?fid=12453.
63. L. Dossey, *ibid.*, pp. 24-27.
64. *Ibid.*, pp. 42-43
65. *Ibid.*, pp. 29-30
66. R. Rosenman, R. Friedman, and M. Friedman, *Type A Behaviour and Your Heart*, 1974, Knopf, New York.
67. See also T. Holmes and R. Rahe, "The Social Readjustment Rating Scale," *Journal of Psychosomatic Research*, 1976, vol. 11, pp. 213-18.
68. M. M. Burg, "Stress, Behaviour and Heart Disease". In G.J. Subak-Sharpe (ed) *Yale University School of Medicine Heart Book, 2002,* Yale University School of Medicine: IAIMS.
69. M. Ferguson, *ibid.*, p. 165
70. Among H. Benson's books on this topic are *The Relaxation Response*, 1975, William Morrow, New York; *The Mind/Body Effect*, 1979, Simon and Schuster, New York; and *Beyond the Relaxation Response* (with W Proctor), *op. cit.*,
71. See, for example, H. Benson, B. A. Rosner, and B. R. Marzetta, "Decreased Systolic Blood Pressure in Hypertensive Subjects Who Practiced Meditation," *Journal of Clinical Investigation*, 1973, vol. 52, p. 8a; R K Wallace, "Physiological Effects of Transcendental Meditation," 1970, *Science*, vol. 167, pp. 1751-54; R K Wallace, " The

Physiology of Meditation," *Scientific American*, 1972, vol. 226. pp. 85-90.
72. Miccozi, *ibid.*

Chapter 4 The theory of transformative subjugation and understanding its ramifications for integrated well-being

1. I. Hacking, "The Disunity of Sciences", in P. Gallison and D. Stump (eds), *The Disunity of Science*, 1996, Stanford University Press, Stanford.
2. J. Rifkin, *Declaration of a Heretic*, 1985, Routledge and Kegan Paul, New York.
3. R.S. Laura and T. Marchant, "Where the mind goes so goes the soul", *Educational Research and Perspectives*,2000, Vol. 27, no. 1., pp. 37-56.
4. R. S. Laura and M. Cotton, *Empathetic Education*, 1999, Falmer Press, Philadelphia.
5. B. T. Hunter, *The Great Nutrition Robbery*, 1978, Scribners, New York, pp. 44-48; see also C. M. Briggs, "Nutritional Aspects of Fabricated Foods," in G. E. Inlgett, ed. *Fabricated Foods*, 1975, AVI Press, Westport, Ct.
6. R. Rodale, "Nutrition: The Historical Imperative," in J. S. Gordon, D. T. Jaffe, and D. E. Bresler, eds., *Mind, Body and Health*, pp. 91-92.
7. see also, L.E. Gross, E.S. Ford, S. Liu, "Increased consumption of refined carbohydrates and the epidemic of type 2 diabetes in the United States: an ecological assessment".2004, *Clin. Nutr.* 2004 May; vol. 79, no. 5, pp 774-779.
8. T. L. Cleve, *The Saccharine Disease*, 1975, Keats Press, New Canaan, Ct., pp. 44-48.
9. J. Fadiman, "Food and Nutrition," in A. C. Hastings, J. Fadiman, and J.S. Gordon, eds., *Health for the Whole Person*, pp. 248-249.
10. see also, Harris R. "Grains, Breakfast Cereals and Bread" in Harris R. *Slim Forever*.2002, London, Sunshine Publications.
11. R. H. Hall, *Food for Thought: The Decline of Nutrition*, 1976, Random House, New York, pp. 106-110.
12. D.S. Smith, J.N.Cash, W. Nip and Y.H. Hui, *Processing Vegetables: Science and Technology*, 1997, CRC Press.
13. Illinois Department of Public Health. Salmonella; c2000-2008 Cited August 2008, http://www.idph.state.il.us/public/hb/hbsam.htm E: see also M. Mellon, C. Benbrook, K.L. Brenbrook, *Estimates of Antimicrobial Abuse in livestock.* Union of Concerned Scientists, 2001 January.
14. *Ibid.*
15. "Secretary's Commission on Pesticides and Their Relationship to Environmental Health," *Report to The Secretary's Commission*,

December, 1969, U.S. Department of Health, Education and Welfare, Washignton, D.C.

16. We wish to express our gratitude to Mr. John F. Ashton, Chief Chemist, Australasian Food Laboratories, for generously permitting some of his collaborative research with Professor R S Laura to be summarised here. For a full account of the health issues involving chlorination see, J. F. Ashton and R. S. Laura, "A Hundred Years of Water Chlorination: Towards a Second of Misgivings," 1989, *Ultra-Health*, vol. 2, no. 2, pp. 52-68.
17. L. Hodges, *Environmental Pollution*, 1977, Holt, Rinehart and Winston, New York, p. 189.
18. W J Llewellyn, "Letter to the Editor," *Journal of American Medical Association*, 1951, vol. 146, no. 13, p. 1273
19. *Ibid.*
20. H. M. Sinclair, cited by L. Clark in *Get Well Naturally*, 1971, ARC Books, New York, p. 327.
21. R. A. Passwater, *Super-Nutrition for Health Hearts*, 1978, Jove Publications, New York, p. 155.
22. *Ibid.*
23. *Ibid*, p. 156.
24. J. M. Price, *Coronaries, Cholesterol, Chlorine*, 1984, Pyramid Publications, Banhadlog Hall, Llanridloes, pp 32-33.
25. E. .P Benditt, "Atherosclerosis May Start with Cell Proliferation," 1974, vol. 227, no. 7, p. 734.
26. N. W. Revis, P. McCauley, R. Bull, and G. Holdsworth, "Relationship of Drinking Water Disinfectants to Plasma Cholesterol and Thyroid Hormone Levels in Experimental Studies," *Proceedings of the National Academy of Science*, March 1986, vol. 83, p. 1485.
27. *Ibid.*, p. 1489
28. "Preliminary Assessment of Suspected Carcinogens in Drinking Water," *Report to Congress*, 1975, U.S. Environmental Protection Agency, Washington, D.C.
29. "Water Contaminated Throughout U.S.," *Chem & Eng. News*, April 28, 1975, p. 19.
30. B. Dowty, D. Carlisle, and J. . Laseter, "Halogenated Hydrocarbons in New Orleans Drinking Water and Blood Plasma," *Science*, 1975, vol. 187, pp. 75-77.
31. T. Page, R. H. Harris, and S. S. Epstein, "Drinking Water and Cancer Mortality in Louisiana," *Science*, 1976, vol. 193, pp. 55-57.
32. See, for example, M. J. Trehy and T. I. Bieber, "Detection, Identification and Quantitative Analysis of Dihalocetonitriles in Chlorinated Natural Waters," L. H. Klein, ed., *Advances in Identification and Analysis of Organic Pollutants in Water*, 1981, Ann Arbor Science Pub., Ann Arbor, Mi., pp. 932-44; see also A. Bruchet et. al., "Characterisation of Total Halogenated Compounds During Various Water Treatment Processes in Water Chlorination," *Chemistry*

Environmental Impact and Health Effects, vol. 5, 1984, Lewis Publisher, Michigan, pp. 1160-74.

33. M. K. Smith et. al., "Developmental Toxicity of Halogenated Acentontriles: Drinking Water By-Products of Chlorine Disinfection," *Toxicology*, 1987, vol. 46, pp 83-93.
34. see also T.J. Doyle,W. Zheng, J.R.Cerhan, C.P Hong, T.A. Sellers, L.H. Kushi and A.R Folsom, "The association of drinking water source and chlorination by-products with cancer incidence among postmenopausal women in Iowa: a prospective cohort study." 1997 *Am J Pub Health*, vol. 87, no. 7, pp 1168-1176.
35. see also J.K. Jouni, A. Skrondal , A. Alexander, G. Becker, T. Krogh and E. Dybing, "Water Chlorination and Birth Defects", 2000, *Obstetrical and Gynecological Survey*"., March vol. 55, no. 3, pp 134-135.
36. For a comprehensive account of the fluoridation controversy, see R. S. Laura and J. F. Ashton, "The Great Flouridation Hoax: Fact or Fiction?" *Nature and Health*, 1989, vol. 11, no. 1, pp 24-40; .J F. Ashton and R. S. Laura, "A Hundred Years of Water Chlorination," *Nature and Health*, vol. 10, no. 4, 1988, pp 44-49.
37. D. Stevenson, "Flouridation Panacea or Poison? *Simply Living*, 1988, vol. 3, no. 6, p. 102.
38. G. Caldwell and P. E. Zanfagna, *Flouridation and Truth Decay*, Top-Ecol Press, Van Owen Reseda, Ca., 1974.
39. G. S. R. Walker, *Flouridation Poison on Tap*, Glen Walker Publisher, Melbourne, 1982, p. 40.
40. *Ibid.*
41. *Ibid.*, p. 156.
42. S. Erbacher, "The Fluoride Debate-Are We Poisoning Our Children?", 2008, *Kindred*, vol. 25, pp 46-48.
43. *D. Stevenson, Ibid.*, p. 104
44. C. Bryson, *The Fluoride Deception*, 2004, New York, Seven Stories Press.
45. J. Mann, M. Tibi, and H. D. Sgan-Cohen, "Fluorosis and Caries Prevalence in a Community Drinking Above-Optional Fluoridated Water," *Community Dent. Oral Epidemiol.*, 1987, vol. 15, pp. 293-95.
46. Erbacher, *ibid.*
47. *Ibid.*
48. A. Howard, *An Agricultural Testament*,1943, Oxford University Press, New York.
49. E.R. Riegel, *Industrial Chemistry*,1937, Reinhold, New York.
50. *Ibid.*, p.149.
51. F. Graham, *Since Silent Spring*, 1970, Hamish Hamilton, London.
52. R. Edwards, "Tomorrow's bitter harvest", 1996, 17th August.
53. See for example, *Alternative Agriculture*, 1989, pp. 40-48.
54. L. Wickenden, *Our Daily Poison*,1961, Hillman Books, New York, p.36.

55. Howard, *ibid.,* 1943, p.30
56. *Ibid.,* p.19.
57. B.C. Nicholson, *Australian Water Quality Criteria for Organic Compounds*, Australian Water Resource Council Technical Paper 82, 1984, pp.214-215.
58. The Conservation Foundation, *State of Environment: A View Towards the Nineties*, 1987,The Conservation Foundation, Washington D.C., p.351,
59. *Ibid*, p.146.
60. *Ibid*,. p.350.
61. *Ibid,* p.352.
62. J. Reisner, "Nader's new beef", *Food Business*, 1989, 5th June, p.30.
63. Carson, *ibid.,*pp. 218-222.
64. S.K. Nigam and A.B. Karnik, "Experimental and human surveillance on BHC and DDT insecticides commonly used in India", *Annals of the New York Academy of Science*, no.534, p.694.
65. Howard, *ibid.,* pp.171-180.
66. See for example, R. Taylor and M.J. Nobbs, *Hunza the Himalayan Shangri-La*, 1962, California: Whitehorn Publishing Co.
67. E.G. Toomey & P.D. White, "A brief survey of the health of aged Hunzas", *American Heart Journal,* 1964, vol. 68, no. 6., pp. 841-842.
68. S. Hedges, "Compost is a natural-born killer", New Scientist, 1996, 21st September, p. 25.
69. J. Seymour, "Hungry for a new revolution", New Scientist, 1996, 30th March, pp.32-37.
70. D. Pimental and C.A. Edwards, "Pesticides and ecosystems*", Bio Science*, 1982, no.32, pp. 595-600.
71. J.R. Smith, *Tree Crops: A Permanent Agriculture,* 1977, Devin-Adair Co, Old Greenwich.
72. I. Anderson, "Australia's Growing Disaster, *New Scientist,*1995, 29th July, no.147, pp.12-13.
73. The Conservation Foundation, *ibid.,* pp.99-109.
74. *Ibid*., p. 351.
75. O. Strebel, W.H.M.Duynisveld and J. Bottcher, "Nitrate pollution of ground-water in Western Europe", *Agricultural Ecosystems and Environment,* 1989, no. 26, pp. 189-214.
76. G. R. Conway and J.N. Petty, "Fertilizer risks in the developing countries", *Nature*, 1988, 21st July, pp.207-208.
77. S. Pain, "Pollutants collect on continental side of North Sea, study finds", *New Scientist,* 1989, 11th November, p. 6.
78. J. E. Krumm, "Fitness Insurance," *Muscle and Fitness*, 1987, vol. 46, no. 10, pp. 11ff.
79. R. Rodale, *op. cit*., p. 90.
80. See, for example, R. S. Laura, "Exercise, Fitness and Health," *Australia Fitness and Training*, 1988 Annual, pp. 8-13.
81. *Ibid*., pp. 9-10..

82. *Ibid.*, pp. 12-13.
83. C.Morris and S. Carson, "Routine Vitamin Supplementation to Prevent Cardiovascular Disease", *Ann Intern Med*, 2003, vol. 139, no. 1, pp 56-70.
84. L. Lamb, "Heart Attacks and Strokes," *Muscle and Facilities*, 1988, vol. 49, no. 2, pp. 80ff.
85. R .S. Parffenbarger, Jr and W. E. Hale, "Work Activity and Coronary Heart Disease," *New England Journal of Medicine*, 1976, vol. 292, pp. 545-50; see also R. S. Parffenberger, Jr, A. L. Wing, and R. T. Hyde, "Contemporary Physical Activity and Incidence of Heart Attack in College Men," *Circulation*, 1977, vol. 56, pp. 3-15 (Abstract); see also R. S. Parffenberger, Jr, W. E. Hale, R. J. Brand and R. T. Hyde, "Work Energy Level, Personal Characteristics, and Fatal Heart Attack," *American Journal of Epidemiology*, 1977, vol. 105, pp. 200-13.
86. P. Kokkinos, J. Myers, J.P. Kokkinos, et al., ''Exercise capacity and mortality in black and white men," *Circulation,* 2008, vol. 107, pp 734-764.
87. Department of Health and Human Services, Centre for Disease and Control. "Basic Statistics. c2008," cited August 2008, www.cdc.gov/topics/surveillance/basic.htm.
88. Ibid.
89. O. C. Simonton & S .Matthews-Simonton, "A Psychphysiological Model for Intervention in the Treatment of Cancer," in J. S. Gordon, D. T .Jaffe, and D. E. Bresler, eds., *Mind, Body, and Health*, pp. 146-63.
90. The University of Texas MD Anderson Medical Centre, "Just the Facts....Smoking and Tobacco Use. c2004, cited March 2008, http://www.mdanderson.org/pdf/pued_smoking.pdf
91. R. S. Laura, "Exercise, Diet and Cancer," *Nature and Health*, 1989, vol. 11, no. 3, pp 44-49.
92. J. Branium "Bodybuilding, Nutrition and Cancer" *op. cit.*, p. 85.
93. *Ibid.*
94. *Ibid.*
95. E. Calle, C. Rodriguez, K. Thurmond, M. Thun, "Overweight, Obesity and Mortality from Cancer in a Prospectively Studied Cohort of US Adults", 2003, *N Eng J Med*, vol. 348, pp 1625-1638.
96. See T Kostrubala, *The Joy of Running*, Pocket Books, New York, 1977, pp. 94ff.
97. S. Biddle, K. Fox, & S. Boutcher, *Physical Activity and Psychological Well-being,* 2000, Routledge, New York.
98. A. Maslow, *Towards a Psychology of Being*, 2d ed., Van Nostrand, Princeton, 1968, p. 55.
99. World Health Organisation, "Australia's disturbing health disparities set Aboriginals apart", *Bulletin of the World Health Organisation*, 2004, vol. 86, no.4, pp 241-320.
100. World Health Organisation, *Targets for Health for All 2000*, 1986, European Regional Office, Copenhagen, p. 17

101. United Nations Department of Public Information, "Supplying water for a price", 2003.
102. R. Philips, "How much 'aid' will reach the tsunami survivors" C1998-2008, cited January 2008, http://www.wsws.org/articles/2005/jan2005/tsun-j11.shtml
103. S. N. Banoub, "No Health for All without Peace for All," *World Health Forum*, 1986, vol. 7, p. 88.
104. T. Solantus et. al., "The Threat of War in the Minds of 12-18 Year Olds in Finland," *The Lancet*, 1984, vol. 8330, no. 1, pp. 784-785.
105. S. N. Banoub, *ibid.*, p. 88.

Chapter 5 From the individual to the social body: Community as good medicine

1. K. C. Tang, R. Beaglehole & E. de Leeuw E (eds) *Health Promotion International 2005: Proceedings of the 6th Global Conference on Health Promotion Bangkok,* Thailand, 2007, International Union for Health Promotion and Education, Oxford University.
2. J. F. March, Global Health: A Gordian knot, 2008, cited June 2008, from http://www.medicc.org/ns/index.php?s=13&p=0
3. B M Kleczkowski, "Matching Goals and Health Care Systems: An International Perspective," *Social Science and Medicine*, 1982, p. 14A, p. 392.
4. World Health Organisation, *Health for All Series*, 1985, no. 9, p. 10.
5. J Fry, *Primary Car*, Heinman Books, London, 1980, p. vii.
6. S. Litsios, "Primary Health Care and Adult Education: Opportunities for Joining Forces," *Convergance*, 1982, vol. xv, no. 2, p. 14.
7. Fry, *ibid.*
8. D. E. Rogers, "The Challenge of Primary Health Care," *Daedalus*, 1977, vol. 106, pp. 81-103.
9. Fry, *ibid.*
10. WHO, *ibid.*, p. 12.
11. *Ibid.*, p. 14.
12. WHO, *Health for All Series*, 1985, no. 1, p. 37.
13. Fry, *ibid.*, p. 519.
14. Joint Commission Public Policy Symposium, *Overuse, Underuse, Misuse: Reducing Waste and Improving efficiency in Health Care*, 2008, Chicago, U.S. Joint Commission Resources.
15. S. I. Benn, Justice in P. Edwards, (ed.), *The Encyclopedia of Philosophy*, Macmillan, New York, 1972, p. 298.
16. J. Rawls, *A Theory of Justice*, Oxford University Press, Oxford, 1980, p. 316.
17. Among those health professionals who have considered Rawlsian concepts in relation to health care are J. H. Bryant, S. Kelman, and M .M .Stewart, whose deliberations can be found in *International Journal of Health Services*, 1977, vol. 7, no. 4.

18. Among those who have detracted from Rawls' work are D. L. Schaefer, *Justice or Tyranny? A Critique of John Rawls' Theory of Justice*, National University Publication, Kennikat Press, Port Washington, N.Y., 1979 and R .P. Wolff, *Understanding Rawls: A Reconstruction and Critique of a Theory of Justice*. Princeton University Press, Princeton, N.J., 1977.
19. Rawls, *ibid.*, p. 303.
20. J. H. Bryant, "Principles of Justice as a Basis of Conceptualising the Health Care System," *International Journal of Health Services*, 1977, vol. 7, no. 4, p. 709.
21. M. M. Stewart, "Problems in Applying Principles of Justice to Health Care Systems," *International Journal of Health Services*, 1977, vol. 7, no. 4, pp. 727-31.
22. Bryant, *ibid.*, pp. 737-39.
23. Benn, *ibid.*, p. 298.
24. Spengler's thoughts on rights and responsibilities are well documented in E. J. Schuster, *Human Rights Today: Revolution or Evolution*, Philosophical Library, New York, 1981, p. 99.
25. Thoughts on rights and responsibilities have been collected into one volume UNESCO *Human Rights*, ed. by Sir Julian Huxley, Columbia University Press, New York, 1973.
26. J. D. Colman, "National Health Goals and Objectives" (speech delivered to National Health Forum, Chicago, Illinois, March 20, 1967) quoted in V. R. Fuchs, *Who Shall Live? Health, Economics and Social Choice*, Harper Porch Books, New York, 1983, p. 28.
27. V. R. Fuchs, *ibid.*, p. 38.
28. M. K. Duval, "The Provider, the Government and the Consumer," in J. Knowles, *Doing Better Feeling Worse*, WW Norton & Co., New York, 1977.
29. Fuchs, *ibid.*, p. 28.
30. Fuchs, *ibid.*, p. 29.
31. J. Knowles, *Doing Better Feeling Worse, ibid.*
32. I. Illich, *Medical Nemesis: The Expropriation of Health*, Calder & Boyers, London, 1975, p. 17.
33. Illich, *ibid.*, p. 41.
34. *Ibid.*, p. 166.
35. Better Health Commission Report, *Looking Forward to Better Health*, AGPS, Canberra, 1986, vol. 1, p. 46.
36. Knowles, *ibid.*, p. 80.
37. M. Keller, "Toward a Definition of Health," *Advances in Nursing Science*, 1981, vol. 4, no. 1, pp. 43-51.
38. Cited in Keller, *ibid.*, pp. 49-50.
39. R. Crawford, "You Are Dangerous to Your Health: The Ideology of Victim Blaming," *International Journal of Health Services*, 1977, vol. 7, no. 4, pp. 663-79.

40. D. Wikler, "Who Should Be Blamed For Being Sick," *Health Education Quarterly*, 1987, vol. 14, no. 1, p. 24.
41. Knowles cited in Crawford, *ibid.*, p. 663.
42. Wynder cited on Crawford, *ibid.*, p. 664.
43. McNerney cited in Crawford, *ibid.*, p. 664.
44. J. Eyre, "Economy, Medicine, Health," *International Journal of Health Services*, 1977, vol. 7, no. 1, pp. 1-150.
45. R. Crawford, "A Cultural Account of 'Health': Control, Release, and the Social Body," in J. B. McKinlay, ed., *Issues in the Political Economy of Health Care*, 1984, p. 66.
46. S. Heaney, G. Allen, S. McBay, et. al., " Lay Perceptions of Health: A Starting Point for Health Promotion" (in press).
47. Crawford, *ibid.*, 1984, p. 70.
48. Crawford, *ibid.*, 1984, p. 81.
49. See also J. Brosschot, W. Gerin & J.Thayer, The perseverative cognition hypothesis: A review of worry, prolonged stress-related physiological activation, and health. *Journal of Psychosomatic Research*, 2006, vol.60, no. 2, pp113-124.
50. *Crawford, Ibid.*, 1984, p. 92.
51. *Ibid.*, 1984, p. 97.
52. *Crawford, Ibid.*, 1977.

Chapter 6 People Empowerment: Education for health VS health education

1. J Rogers, cited in R E Kime, et. Al., *Health Instruction: An Action Approach*, Prentice-Hall, New Jersey, 1977, p. 25.
2. E Hartwell, cited in Kime, *ibid.*, p. 26.
3. C Mayshark, "A Descriptive and Comparative Study of the Administrative Patterns Operative in Six School Health Programs," *U.S. Education Office Project 6-8288*, University of Tennessee, Knoxville, 1967.
4. K L Lorig and J Laurin, "Some Notions about Assumptions Underlying Health Education," *Health Education Quarterly*, 1985, vol. 10, no. 3, pp. 231-43.
5. "Multiple Risk Factor Intervention Trial," *Journal of the American Medical Association*, 1982, vol. 248, pp. 1465-77.
6. *Ibid.*, p. 1466.
7. R Paffenberger et. al., "Work Energy Level, Personal Characteristics and Fatal heart Attack: A Birth Cohort Effect," *American Journal of Epidemiology*, 1977, vol., 108, pp. 161-75.
8. A W Sedgewick, et. al., "Long-Term Effects of Physical Training Programme on Risk Factors for Coronary Disease in Otherwise Sedentary Men," *British Medical Journal*, 1980, vol. 281, pp. 7-10.
9. P Puska et. al., "Changes in Coronary Risk Factor during a Comprehensive Five-Year Community Programme to Control

Cardiovascular Disease. (North Karelia Project)," *British Medical Journal*, 1979, vol. 2, pp. 1173-77.

10. J T Salonen et. al., "Changes in Morbidity and Mortality during Comprehensive Community Programme to Control Cardiovascular Disease during 1972-1977 in North Karelia," *British Medical Journal*, 1979, vol. 2, pp. 1178-83.
11. K Koskela et. al., "Changes in Cardiovascular Disease-Related Health Behaviour during Ten Years of Preventive Community Program," *Stanford University Health Research Seminar*, Dec. 12th, 1983.
12. D. Leyden et al., "Teaching Behavioural Medicine using Individual Coronary Heart Disease Risk factors", *Preventative Medicine*, 1987, vol. 16, pp.269-73.
13. *Ibid.*, p.273.
14. A. R. Assaf et. al., "Comparison of Three Methods of Teaching Woman How to Perform Breast Self-Examination", *Health Education Quarterly*, 1985, vol.12, no.3, pp.259-272.
15. *Ibid.*, p.271
16. C. Flaherty et. al., "Breast-Screening Clinic Versus Health Education Sessions as Outlets for Education in Breast Self Examination," *Journal of Epidemiology and Community Health*, 1986, vol. 46, pp. 67-70.
17. M. M. Roberts et. al., "Edinburgh Breast Education Campaign on Breast Cancer and Breast Self-Self Examination: Was it Worthwhile?" *Journal of Epidemiology and Community Health*, 1987, vol. 41, pp. 338-343.
18. *Ibid.*, p.343.
19. J. Gravell et. al., "Impact of Breast Self-Examination, Planned Educational messages and Social Network Communications: An Exploratory Study", *Health Education Quarterly*, 1985, vol. 12, no.1, pp. 51-64.
20. B. F. Stanton et.al., "Twenty Four Hour Recall, Knowledge-Attitude-Practice Questionnaire, and Direct Observation of Sanitary Practices. A Comparative Study," *Bulletin of World Health Organization*, 1987, vol.65, no. 2, pp.217-222.
21. P.J. Homel et. al., "Effective Health and Personal Development: An Experiment in School Education," *The Medical Journal of Australia*, 1982, July 10, pp. 41-42.
22. *Ibid.*, p.42.
23. M. N. Maddock et. al., "Attitude to Health and Knowledge of Health Issues in Nurses, High School and Primary School Pupils", *Research in Education*, 1984, vol. 14, pp. 14-22.
24. G. S. Parcel et. al., "Preschool Health Education Program (PHEP): Analysis of Educational and Behavioural Outcomes," *Health Education Quarterly*, 1984, vol. 10, p.149-172.
25. Homel, *op. cit.*
26. Schoenbach, V., "Appraising health risk appraisal" (editorial), *American Journal of Public Health*, 1987, vol. 77, pp.409-411.

27. P Berry, W Schoenbach, V Wagner, E.M Graham, R.Karon, & S Pezzullo, *Health Risk Appraisal: Methods and Programs with Annotated Bibliography*, National Centre for Health Services Research and Health Care Technology, 1986, Washington, DC.
28. J. M. McKenny et. al., "The Effect of Clinical Pharmacy Services on Patients with Essential Hypertension", *Circulation*, 1973, vol 140.86, pp.646-651.
29. T. S. Inui et. al., "Improving Outcomes in Hypertension after Physician Tutorial: A Controlled Trial," *Annuals of Internal Medicine*, 1976, vol.86, pp.646-651.
30. D. G. Nessman et.al., "Increasing Compliance. Patient Operated Hypertension Groups," *Archives of Internal Medicine*, 1980, vol. 140, pp.1427-1430.
31. R. B. Haynes et. al., Improvement in Medication Compliance in Uncontrolled Hypertension , *Lance*t, 1976, vol. 1, pp.1265-1268.
32. D. E. Morisky et. al., "Evaluation of Family Health Education to Build Social Support for Long Term Control of Blood Pressure", *Health Education Quarterly*, 1985, vol. 12, no. 1, pp.35-50.
33. T.F. William, D. A Martin, M. D. Hogan et. al., "The clinical picture of diabetic control studied in four setting," *American Journal of Public Health*, 1967, vol. 57, pp.441-451.
34. K.L. Webb et. al., "Evaluation of a Diabetes Education Program", *Australia New Zealand Journal of Medicine*, 1982, vol. 12, pp.153-159.
35. F. W. Whitehouse et.al., "Teaching the Person with Diabetes: Experience with a Follow-Up Session," *Diabetes Care*, 1979, vol. 2, no.1, pp.35-38.
36. Brownell cited in Lorig and Laurin, *op. cit*., p.236.
37. P.M. Stanlonas et. al., Behaviour Modification for Obesity: The Evaluation of Exercise Contingency Management and Program Adherence, "Journal of Consultant and Clinical Psychology, 1978, vol. 46, no. 3, pp. 463-469.
38. R.F. Kushner, "Barriers to providing nutritional counselling by physicians: a survey of primary care practioners", *Prev Med*, 1995, vol. 24, pp.546-552.
39. M.H. Liang et.al., "Design and Evaluation of a Pilot Community Programme for Musculoskeletal Disability", *Journal of Community Health*, 1981, vol. 4, no. 3, pp.257-266.
40. M. Potts and K. Brandt, "Analysis of Education Support Groups for Patients with Rheumatoid Arthritis," *Patient Counsel Health Education*, 1983, vol. 4, no. 30, pp.161-166.
41. K.L. Lorig et. al., "on Association Between Improved Arthritis Health Behaviour and Health Status: A Possible Explanatory Hypothesis", *Arthritis Rheumatology*, 1984, vol. 26, no. 5, pp. 54-56.
42. Ibid
43. A Eagly & S Chaiken, *The Psychology of Attitudes*, Harcourt Brace & Company, Florida, 1993.

44. J. B. Rotter, *Social Learning and Clinical Psychology*, 1954, Prentice Hall, Englewood Cliffs, N.J.
45. A. Bandura et. al., "Relative Efficiency of Dissemination and Modelling Therapeutic Approaches for Inducing Behavioural, Affective and Attitude Changes", *Journal of Personal Psychology*, 1969, vol. 13, pp. 173-179.
46. A. Bandura, Efficacy of Participant Modelling as a Function of Response Induction Aids," Journal of Abnormal Psychology, 1969, vol. 13, pp.173-179.
47. A. Bandura, "Self Efficacy: Toward a Unifying Theory of Behaviour Change," *Psychology Review*, 1977, vol. 84, pp. 191-215.
48. A. Bandura, "Self-Efficacy Mechanism in Human Agency." *American Journal of Psychology*, 1982, vol. 2, pp. 122-147.
49. E. P. Bettinghaus, "Health Promotion and Knowledge-Attitude-Behaviour Continuum", *Preventative Medicine*, 1986, vol. 15, pp. 475-491.
50. I. Rosenstock, "The Health Belief Model and Preventative Health Behaviour," Health Education Monographs, 1972, vol. 2, no. 4, pp.254-386.
51. R. S. Downie & C. Fyfe, "Health Education in Schools" in S. Doxiadis ed., *Ethics in Health Education*, 1990, Wiley, Chichester.
52. E. G. Boring, *A History of Experimental Psychology, 1950*, Appleton Century Crofts, New York.
53. B. F. Skinner, *Beyond Freedom and Dignity*, 1971, A. A. Knopf, New York.
54. R. S Downie & C. Fyfe, *ibid.*
55. J. Dewey cited in Kime, *ibid.*, p.48.
56. H. Taba, *Curriculum Development: Theory and Practice*, 1962, Harcourt, Brace, Jovanovich, New York.
57. Combs cited in Kime, *ibid.*, p.48.
58. D. Callahan & B. Jennings, "Ethics and Public Health: Forging a Strong Relationship," *American Journal of Public Health*, 2002, vol. 92, no.2, pp.169-176.
59. W.K. Frankena, "A Model for Analysing a Philosophy of Education", in J. R. Martin, *Readings in the Philosophy of Education: A Study of Curriculum*, 1970, Allyn & Bacon, Boston.
60. *Ibid.*, p.22.
61. A. Robertson, "Health promotion and the common good: reflections on the politics of need," in D. Callahan, ed., *Promoting healthy behaviour: How much freedom? Whose responsibility?* 2001, Washington D.C. Georgetown University Press, pp.76-94.
62. P. Duncan, *Critical Perspectives on Health*, Palgrave MacMillan, New York, 2007
63. R. R. Shrweder, N. C. Munch, M. Mahapatra, & L. Park, L, "The 'big three' of morality (autonomy, community, divinity) and the 'big three'

explanations of suffering", in A.M. Brandt & P. Rosin eds., *Morality and Health,* Routledge, New York, pp. 119-172.

64. M. Blaxter, *Health and Lifestyles*, Routledge, London, 1990.
65. L. Leviton, C. E. Needleman, M.A. & Sharpio,*Confronting Public Health Risks: A Decision Makers Guide*, California, Sage Publication, 1996.
66. P. Freire, Pedagogy of the Oppressed, 1974Seabury Press, New York, p. 46.

Chapter 7 The philosophical principles of unfolding consciousness

1. C. Glymour and D. Stalker, "Quantum Medicine," in *Examining Wwholistic Medicine*, 1980, p. 25.
2. *Ibid.*, p. 26.
3. *Ibid.*, p. 108.
4. *Ibid.*
5. *Ibid.*, p. 109.
6. *Ibid.*, pp. 109-110.
7. *Ibid.*, p. 124.
8. For a more comprehensive account of this description, see R. S. Laura, "Philosophical Foundations of Science Education," *Educational Philosophy and Theory*, 1980, vol. 13, pp. 1-13.
9. This view is elaborated in R. S. Laura, "Wittgenstein's Doctrine of Science: or Does the Philosophical Investigations show less than it says?" *Prudentia*, 1981, Supplementary Number, pp. 153-64.
10. For the elaboration of this view, see W. V. Quine and J. S .Ullian, *The Web of Belief*, 1970, Random House, New York.
11. K. Klein, *Positivism and Christianity*, 1974, M Nijhof, The Hague, pp. 58ff.
12. P. K Feyerbend, *Science in a Free Society*, 1978, New Left Books, pp. 100ff.
13. N. Malcolm, *Ludwig Wittgenstein: A Memoir*, 1958, Oxford University Press, London, p. 88.
14. For the elaboration of this view see R. S. Laura, "Philosophical Foundations of Religious Education," *Educational Theory*, vol. 28, Fall, 1978, pp. 310-317.
15. See, for example, L. Wittgenstein, *On Certainty*, trans. By D. Paul & G. E. M. Anscombe, (eds). G. E. M. Anscombe & G. H. von Wright, 1969, Basil Blackwell, Oxford, para. 125.

Chapter 8 The quantum connection: Consciousness and the new paradigm of health education

1. J. Bell, "On the Einstein-Podolsky-Rosen Paradox", *Physics*, 1964, vol. I., pp. 195-200.

2. The interpretation of Bell's theorem espoused here has, contrary to Stalker and Glymour, who condemn the interpretation as "incoherent, uninformed, and unintelligent," been seriously proposed by distinguished physicists such as Paul Davies, Alain Aspect, John Wheeler, Sir Rudolph Peierls, and even Bell himself. See, for example, Davies' report of his BBC interview with these physicists in P. Davies, *Superforce*, 1984, Unwin Paperbacks, London, pp. 45-49.
3. See, for example, D. Bohm, *Wholeness and the Implicate Order*, 1980, Routledge & Kegan Paul, London.
4. For a full account of this aspect of Bohm's account see G. Zukav, *the Dancing Wu Li Masters*, 1980, Bantam Books, New York, pp. 305-309.
5. Capra, *ibid.*, 1982, p. 292.
6. See, for example, J. E. Lovelock, *Gaia*, 1979, Oxford University Press, New York, p. IX.
7. *Ibid.*
8. *Ibid.,* pp 13-28.
9. K. Warren and N. Erkal, *Ecofeminism: Woman, Culture and Nature*, 1997, Indiana University Press, Indiana.
10. J .Rifkin, *Declaration of a Heretic*, *op. cit*., p. 11.
11. *Ibid*., p. 84.
12. *Ibid*., p. 26.
13. W. Heisenberg, *Physics and Philosophy*, 1963, Allen & Unwin, London, pp. 52-64.
14. For the elaboration of this view see R S Laura, "To Educate or to Indoctrinate: That Is Still The Question," *Educational Philosophy and Theory*, 1983, vol. 18, pp. 43-55.
15. E. N. Goodman, *Ways of Worldmaking*, 1981, Hackett, Cambridge, pp. 120ff (for further discussions of Goodman's view, see C. Z. Elgin, *With Reference to Reference*, 1983, Hackett, Indianapolis)
16. *Ibid*., p. 120

About the Authors

Professor Ronald S. Laura

Dr Ronald S. Laura was born in Boston and educated at the Universities of Harvard, St John's College Cambridge and Brasenose College Oxford, where he completed his Doctoral Studies. He is Professor in Education at the University of Newcastle, Australia and an elected life-time PERC Fellow at Harvard University. In addition to in excess of 200 scholarly articles, he has also published 30 books including Empathetic Education (1999), Integrating Eastern and Western Traditions in Health (2004) and The New Social Disease: From High Tech Depersonalization to Survival of the Soul (2008). He teaches in both the faculty of Education and Arts, offering subjects in the Philosophy of Education, Philosophy of Medicine and Public Health.

Ms Amy Chapman

Amy Chapman is tutor and qualitative researcher at the University of Newcastle, Australia. She is a qualified journalist and secondary English teacher and has completed a Bachelor of Teaching / Bachelor of Arts (Hons). She is currently writing her Doctoral thesis: 'A Critical Exploration of the Epistemological Foundations of Mental Health and their Implications for Reconceptualizing the Importance of the Role of Teaching.' She is published, has presented research papers nationally and internationally and hopes to continue to explore the philosophical and sociological dimensions of health and education.

Mr Mark Hinchey

Mark Hinchey graduated in 2004 with a double degree in Teaching and PDHPE at the University of Newcastle, Australia. In 2005, he was appointed to the Faculty of PDHPE at Saint Phillips College where he taught for a period of three years. He has recently completed a Masters in Health Education and is currently completing a degree in Naturopathy at the Australian Institute of Applied Sciences in Canberra, Australia.

INDEX